vReiki One

Introduction to
The Reiki Revolution

By
Martyn Pentecost

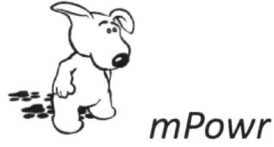

mPowr

First Published in Great Britain 2012 by
mPowr (Publishing) Ltd.
Suite 11352, 2nd Floor, 145–157 St John Street, London EC1V 4PY
www.mpowrpublishing.com
www.mpowrunlimited.com

A catalogue record for this book is available from the British Library
ISBN – 978-1-907282-61-4

Cover Design by Martyn Pentecost
mPowr Publishing 'Clumpy™' Logo by e-nimation.com
Clumpy™ and the Clumpy™ Logo are trademarks of mPowr Ltd.

MADE BY BOOK BROWNIES!

Books published by mPowr Publishing are made by Book Brownies. A Book Brownie is about so high, with little green boots, a potato-like face and big brown eyes. These helpful little creatures tenderly create every book with kindness, care and a little bit of magic! Before shipping, a Book Brownie will jump into the pages—usually at the most gripping chapter or a part that pays particular attention to food—and stay with that book, always. This means that every mPowr Publishing book comes with added enchantment (and occasional chocolate smudges!)

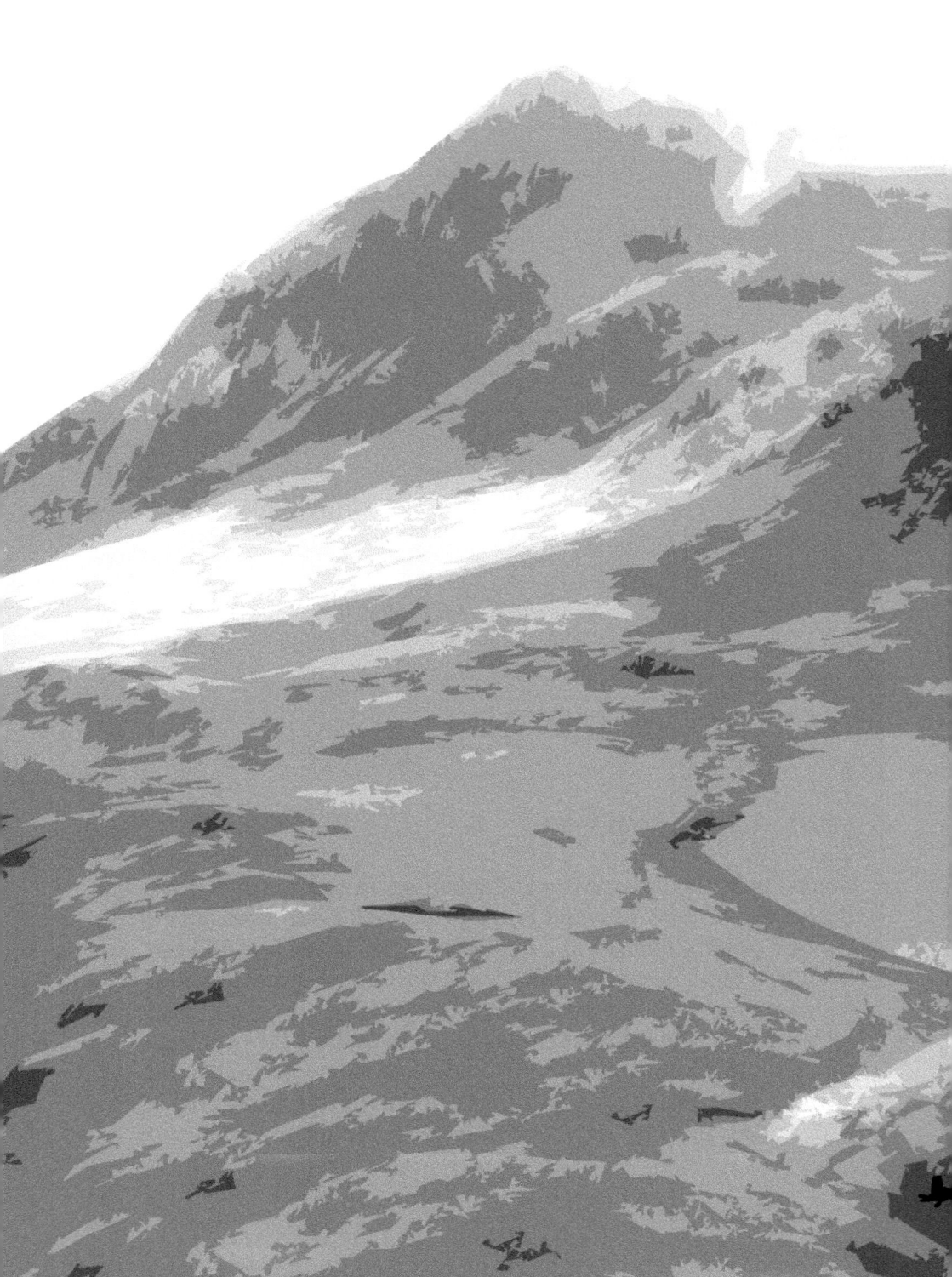

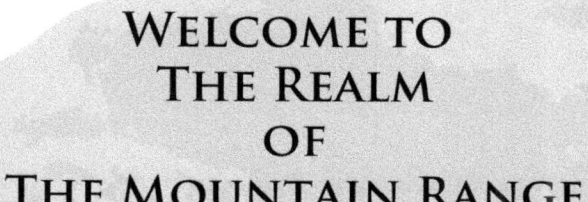

Welcome to
The Realm
of
The Mountain Range

It is in this place,
this Mountain Range,
where we experience our
first glimpse of Ki.
In this place of rock
and air, of thunder and
the moon; here between
the Earth and the sky, we
shall discover a path
that ascends beyond
anything we have
ever known...

Register your copy of this manual to unlock amazing new Realms of Experience. Simply visit *The Reiki Revolution Home Experience* gateway for more information...

http://www.celtic-reiki.com/vreiki/vreikihe.php

Contents

An Introduction to vReiki   11

An Intelligent Force   19

The Ancient Philosophy of Ki   27

Ki and a Modern Reality   37

The History and Development of Usui Reiki   49

Stepping onto the Path   59

A Mysterious Light   75

The Cohesion of Consciousness   81

A Magnetic Power   89

The Dynamics of Intuition   95

The Intuition Workout   105

Appendices   113

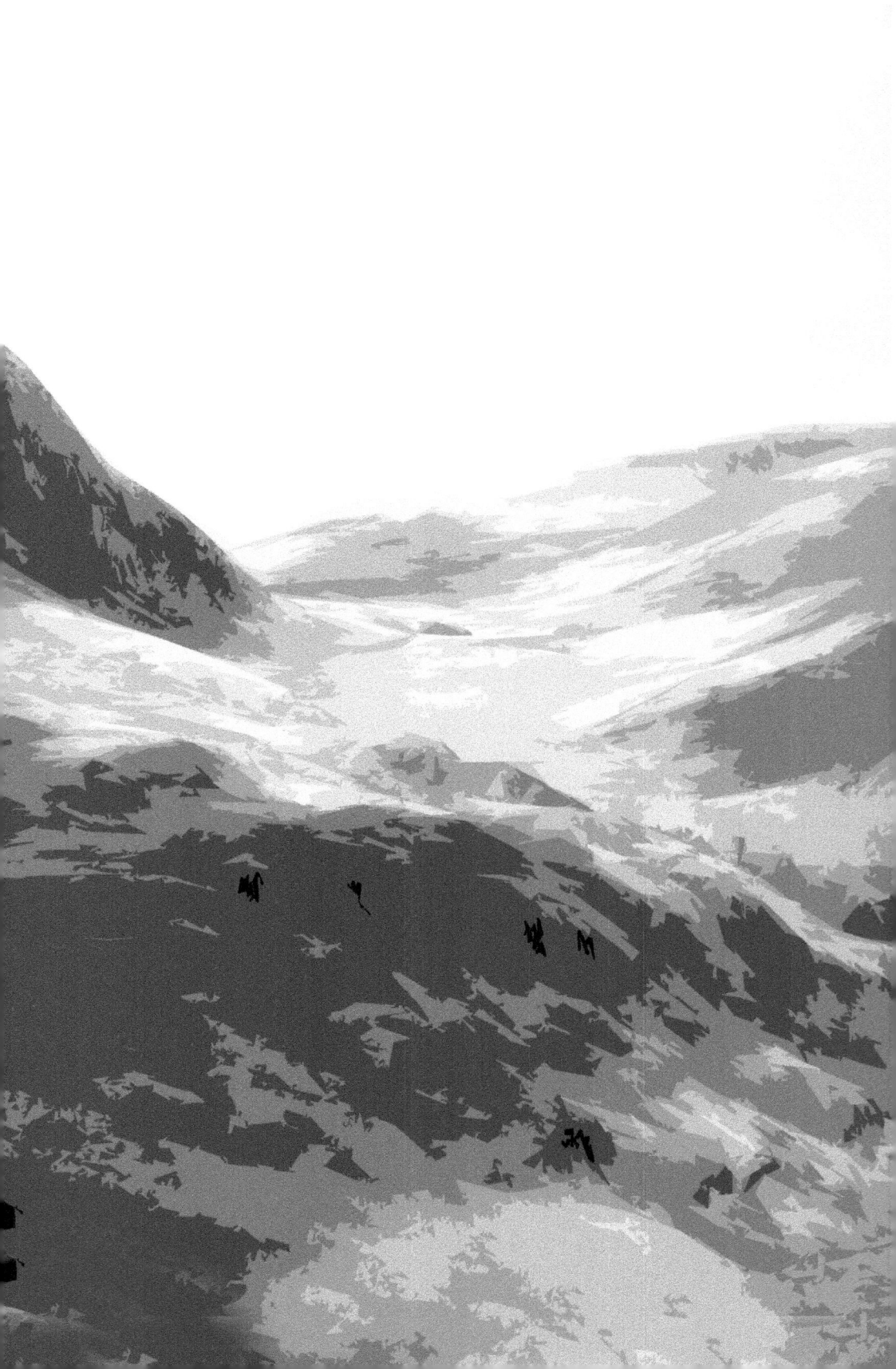

A Revolution Begins...

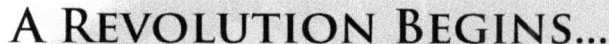

This is a revolution—an uprising—
a total shifting of perspective
from the dogma and cruelty, to
a new sense of compassion and
enlightened dialogue. The way
forward needs strength, courage,
and a proactive approach to stay
on the path.

An Introduction to vReiki

There is an infinite power in the Universe that is intrinsically woven through all things and at all times. This force is innately sentient and is constantly striving to create balance and harmony throughout the incomprehensible complexity that exists all around us and within us. It is a force which has been known for thousands of years as 'Reiki'; the 'Ki' or 'life force' of the Soul.

For many thousands of years, the cultural philosophies that have enabled humankind to understand Reiki have been sufficient enough for people to develop a deep and lasting relationship with this omnipresent, yet elusive power. However, just over a century ago, something happened which set in motion a chain of events; a chain of events that would cause global awareness of Reiki to explode... and to crush the very nature of Reiki simultaneously.

In the early part of the 21st Century, we exist at a time when our awareness of Reiki, and the threads of experience that stem from it, are perilously in the balance. Our actions at this point in time could result in the practices—that are powered by Reiki—becoming an essential aspect of people's lives; helping to heal, strengthen relationships, create success, and develop a deeper sense of compassion and spirituality within us all. Conversely, how we behave at this moment could also obviate Reiki from our consciousness; subjecting those who work with Reiki's magic to bullying, ridicule, and eventually complete obscurity.

We can already see these types of scenarios developing in the communities of Reiki (modality) Masters, where the ego-driven need to be 'right' completely blinds individuals to the damage they inflict. Yet, if we just listen to the messages of Reiki—and beyond this, the source of Reiki—we would evolve a completely new way of communicating our practices to the world and, by doing so, we would unleash even deeper layers of potential for everybody to be immersed in.

Personally, I find discussing this contractive viewpoint of Reiki Mastery very challenging, as I believe this leads to dogma and the desire to disassociate from Reiki practices. Although, on this occasion, I also feel it is a very necessary place to start, because how can we transcend a widespread attitude, without being up front about that attitude?

This is a revolution—an uprising—a total shifting of perspective from the dogma and cruelty, to a new sense of compassion and enlightened dialogue. The way forward needs strength, courage, and a proactive approach to stay on the path. We require advocacy and a sense of legacy to expand onwards, as well as understanding the importance of our community—no one can walk their journey alone, for we are all connected, we are all one.

These principles are reflected in the *Home Experience* you are about to partake in. Presented in a rather unique way, the journey ahead may be very different to what you expect, although the results you achieve along the way will blow your mind!

The way vReiki is presented in this *Home Experience* is with an emphasis on the Traditions of Usui Reiki in the introductory and practitioner degrees. Here we also explore the Viridian philosophies of vReiki (and the Viridian perspective of the other facets of Ki), however, there is a focus on the Usui ethos, because this offers context and contrast. Many people who embark on their vReiki path have previous experience of Usui Reiki and the initial investigation of this modality supports the Apprentice with 'familiar territory'. Even when a person has no Usui Reiki experience, covering these topics at the very beginning of the experience provides any Adventurer of the vReiki path a common tongue, to dialogue with Usui Reiki Masters.

As we progress into the Realms of degrees three and four, the emphasis shifts from Usui Reiki to become entirely about the Viridian perspective of Ki. This modality is totally different from what any Adventurer will be used to (unless they have had previous VM training). For, in Viridian philosophy, we engage with Reiki and the other facets of Ki in a multi-dimensional perspective, where usual attributes of time and space are not only turned on their heads, but also expanded through an elaborate interweaving of science and magic.

In the Mentor and Mastery areas of this *Home Experience*, there is a real sense of Reiki methodology being completely transformed into an art that is very relevant in our technological, scientific, and virtual society—whilst keeping these elements in the background as we focus on the magic and spirituality of our Viridian perspective.

It is important to mention that I do not position Usui Reiki as the 'underdog', or in any way wish to imply that Usui Reiki is a lesser practice. The contextual comparison between Usui and vReiki is essential, because well over a century distances the two modalities (and this was a century where development and change were exponentially greater than at any other time in human history!). By offering both perspectives, my intention is to demonstrate how Reiki modalities are integrally linked to the Age in which they are created.

When tradition is used with respect for the current era and acknowledgement of the challenges faced by our contemporaries, it can work miracles. However, when we cling to tradition as a means to escape the current situations we face (personally, socially, and globally), it becomes dogma — the most detrimental factor that Reiki arts are currently facing. The fact that Usui Reiki Mastery is literally being destroyed by ego is heartbreaking to watch for me, personally. Usui Reiki changed my life... setting me on a path that has taken me all over the world and brought me here to you. To know that for some, the need to be 'right' is more important than the need to empower others is sad, yet this is why vReiki is so powerful. It was originated to offer people a means of discovering their own perspective of Reiki and the modalities we use to interact with it. From the very first moment, you are encouraged to create your own personal relationship with Ki and to express this in your own unique way, whilst respecting the contrast others bring with them.

The Reiki Revolution Home Experience presents this journey of self-discovery in an engaging and extremely enchanting way. The integral connection between these books and the virtual Realm (online), imparts a journey; a magical adventure that immerses you in imagery, music, and narration. A sensory and synaesthetic wonderland, where you can dance, sing, and simply be, whilst you learn amazing abilities.

The nature of the *Home Experience* means that this book is not intended to be read in isolation—in fact, it will not make much sense without the virtual realms—so you are encouraged to interact between the book and virtual realms, in order to fully experience the Realms that exist beyond the *Home Experience*: The Realms within. These are actual 'places' that exist at subtle levels of awareness. To connect to them, explore them, and retain those experiences, we use the Orientation and Calibration processes and the wealth of materials that encourage your connection to the Realms. The books are intended to offer understanding and wisdom; the virtual realms present visual, audio, and synaesthetic triggers to transport you to the 'actual' Realms of vReiki that exist beyond the usual waking consciousness.

As so many of the philosophies and mysticism of vReiki can be intense, the presentation of stories and visual symbolism can help you digest the experience from your own perspective. So, with this in mind, treat the *Home Experience* like an adventure—explore every nook and shadowy corner; lift each stone and dive into every pool; never think that you know what is located in a realm, because you have visited it once (things hide and things change!); be prepared for experiences that contrast with what you are used to, as this is the nature of the *Home Experience*; and finally, treat your journey with child-like wonder... if you approach this path as an adult would, you'll miss the most important messages of all... those that are so sacred, they cannot be written down!

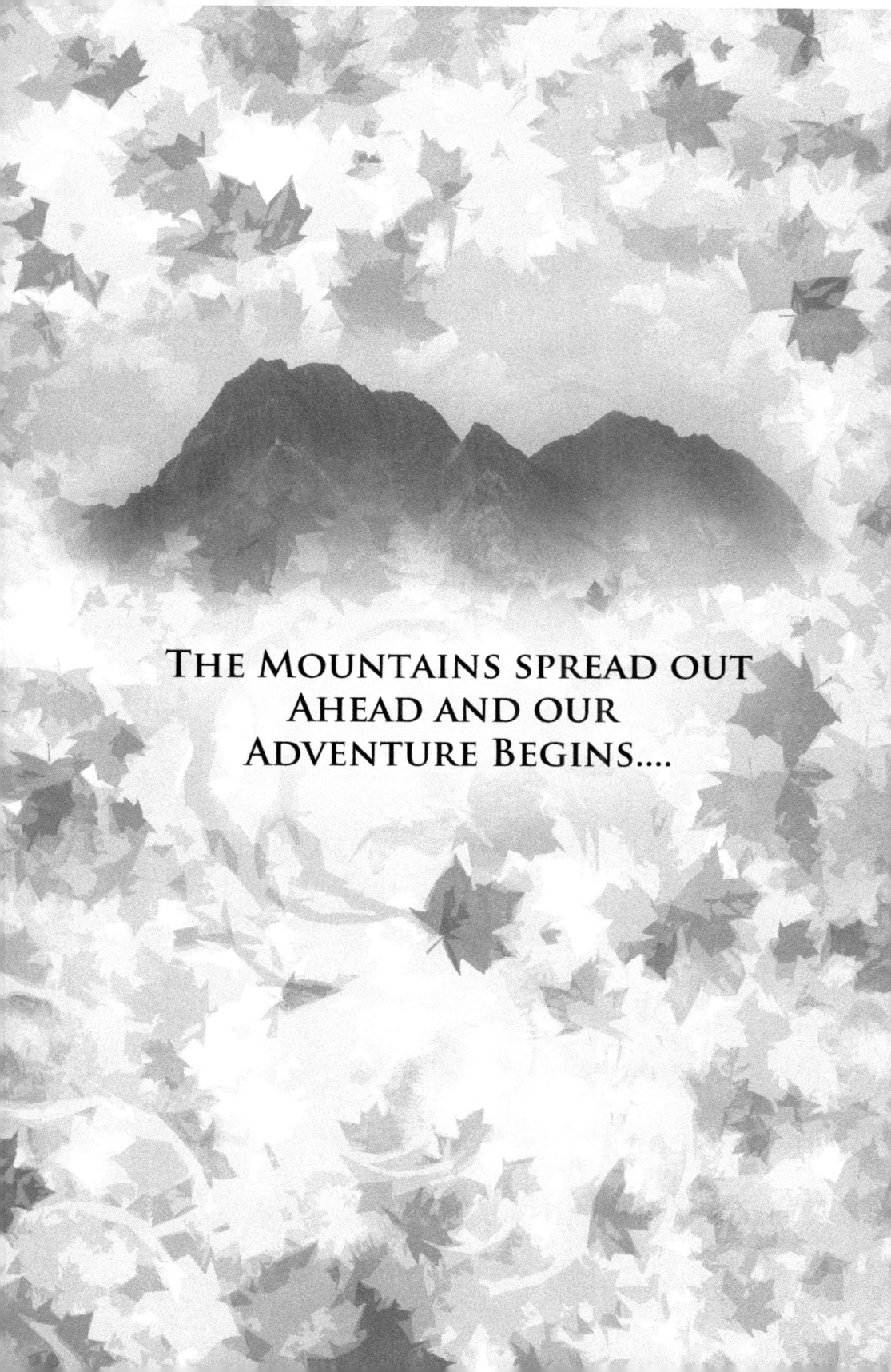

THE MOUNTAINS SPREAD OUT
AHEAD AND OUR
ADVENTURE BEGINS....

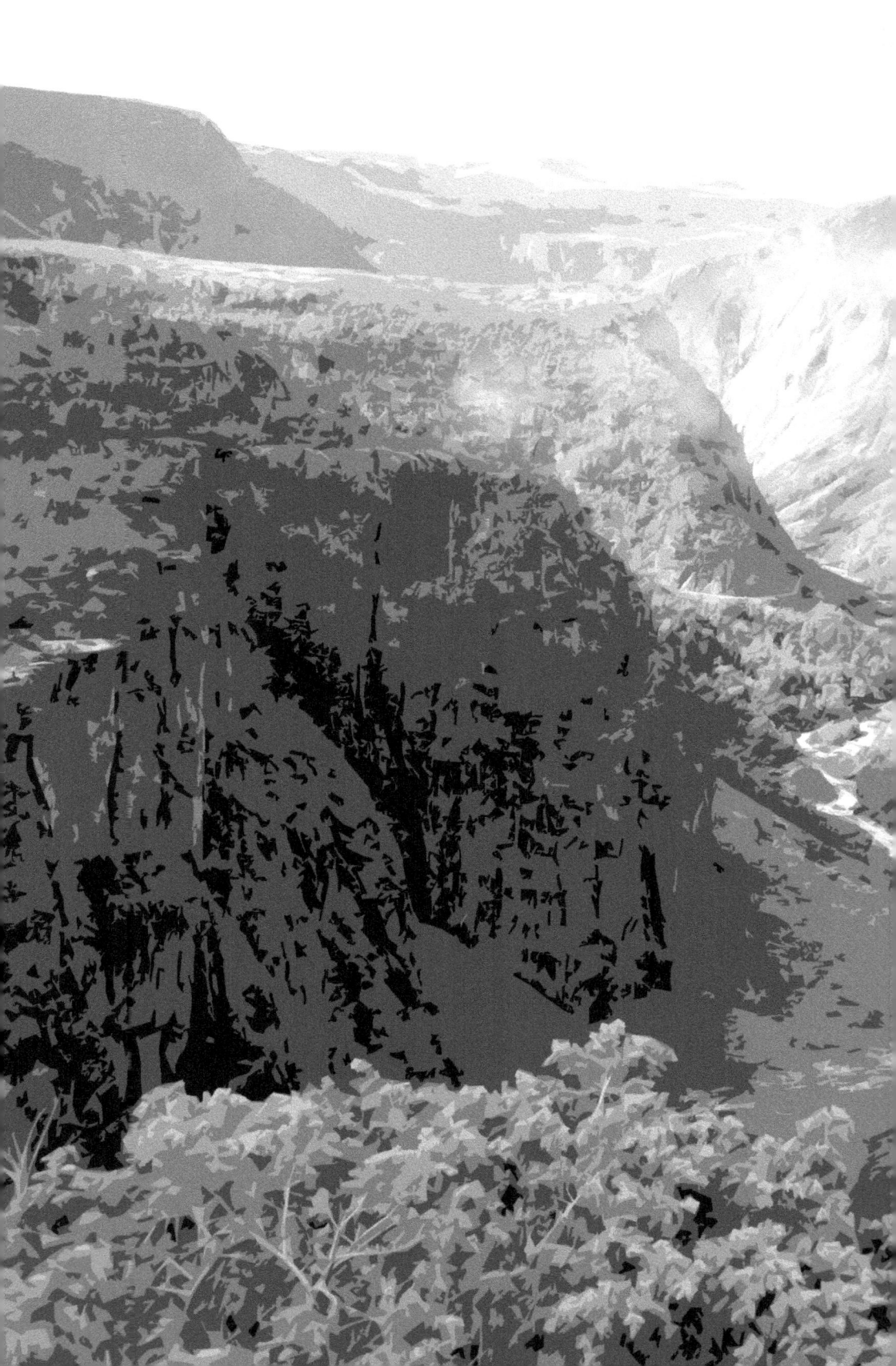

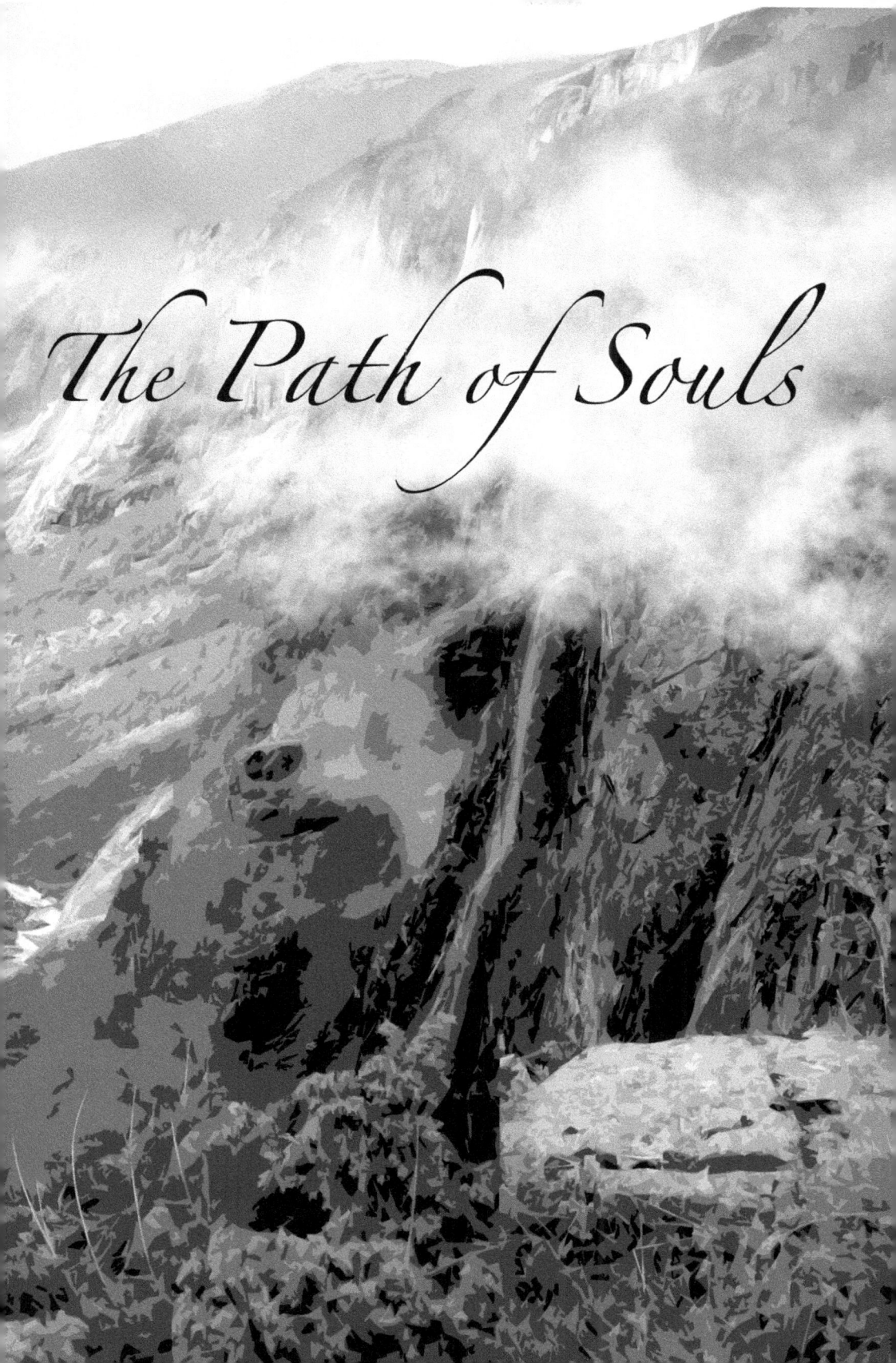

The Path of Souls

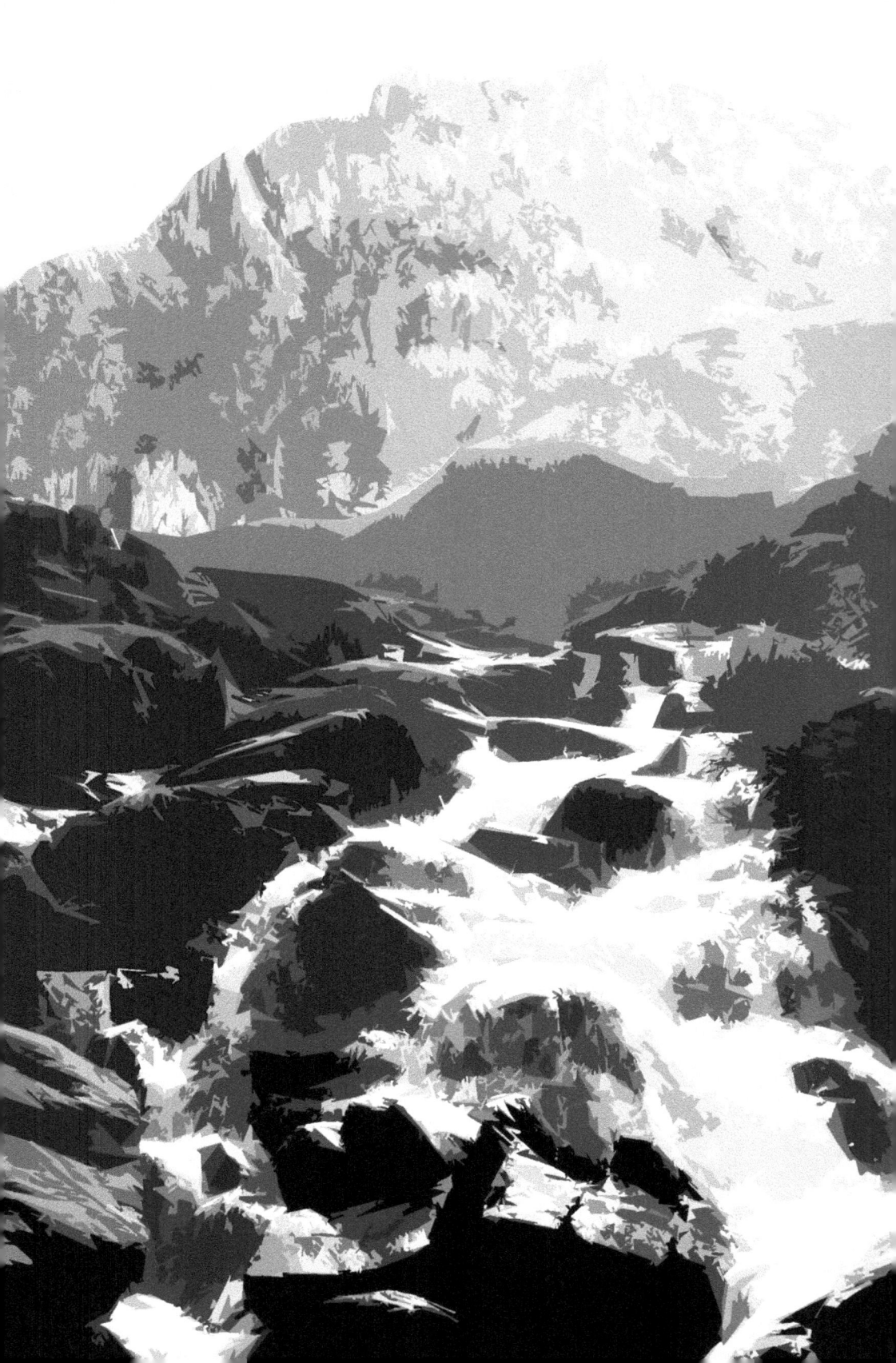

An Intelligent Force

Thought creates the physical world into being. A spark, an idea, a vision can burst into life; transforming the world around us (and within us) in truly miraculous ways. Contrary to popular understanding, thought is not exclusively the function of an individual person, but a transpersonal and Universal phenomenon. Thoughts interweave into complex and sometimes chaotic physicality. The Universe in all its infinite wonder was thought into being, just as people think their lives into reality every day. Indeed, the Viridian philosophies—upon which vReiki is based—state that the creation of the Universe and the thoughts of humankind are actually the same thought, expressed from different perspectives!

For many people, thoughts are what drive us to action, whether this be the need to fulfil desires and dreams, or alleviate fears and worries. Our thoughts influence behaviour, which in turn, creates reality. We literally think our lives into reality before living that reality. The power of thought is so magnificent that people can achieve anything they believe to be possible, regardless of how expansive (or contractive) that belief.

Yet, at an even deeper layer of experience; pure thought and the force encapsulated within that thought, are the essential factors for the physical Universe's very existence. For every thought is like a spark... it has the potential to create a flame. However, when a thought meets some form of contention or opposition, it interacts with the opposing thought to produce physicality. As an interesting aside, many people shy away from resistance or even fear their ideas being opposed—yet it is this very resistance and opposition that facilitates the achievement of their ideas in physical reality.

The force, which is present when two thoughts collide, is the seed of conscious experience. Ancient Shinto philosophy explains that there is a 'trade-off' between intelligence and physicality. Pure intelligence has no physical presence whatsoever and pure physical matter is totally incapable of thought. Yet, between these two polar opposites, exists a whole Universe of wonder and experience and life.

The Shinto concept of Reiki is one of a powerful force that exists in the physical Universe, yet only to a very subtle extent. A tiny proportion of a greater intelligence is exchanged for the least amount of physicality necessary to create change. This puncturing of the physical/non-physical veil is so subtle that the vast majority of people are completely unaware of the existence of Reiki; even fewer consciously experience it with any identifiable form of sensory feedback.

Yet for those of us who do notice the existence of Reiki in our physical Universe, the synaesthesia of our response to it is utterly overwhelming and magical. For there is something deeply instinctual in that interaction; an understanding that two intelligent entities are coming together to create miracles... and that is exactly what we do. As Reiki interacts with another sentient being, the aforementioned change begins to take place: Reiki instils a greater wisdom within us and we present Reiki with our own, unique perspective.

The result of this exchange is often a burst of synaesthesia that can affect us on many different sensory levels. From a visual fireworks display of colour and shape to the most beautiful symphonies of sound. Soaring and indefinable emotions, to feelings of a soothing, internal ebb and flow. Many of these synaesthetic experiences are translated as 'Reiki', yet in my perspective, we are not experiencing 'what Reiki feels or looks like', we are actually reacting to the joy of connection in the same way as a cup of coffee or taste of chocolate can cause a sensory response (albeit with the volume, colour, and kinaesthesia turned to max!).

This belief has created a bit of a storm in the past, because many want to believe the bliss of connection is 'not theirs', i.e.: it is Reiki they are experiencing and not 'just other' internal sensation. The important factor to remember is that *we are actually experiencing Reiki*—our own unique interpretation of it, or what I call 'our perspective of Reiki'. It is your perspective of Reiki that will create the basis of your vReiki Mastery... in other words, a vReiki Master originates their very own practice, based upon their unique perspective and experience.

So, why do we have these synaesthetic reactions to a connection with Reiki, what causes them, and how can we use these experiences to create change?

Reiki is a force—in modern terms, we use the word 'energy'—that has subtle physicality. The nature of Reiki is infinite and it exists at every point in the Universe and at every moment that has ever been, is, or will be. Reiki literally transcends time and space! When we shift our conscious focus to Calibrate to Reiki, we are not 'going anywhere' and Reiki is not 'coming to us', it is merely an acknowledgement that we already exist in the same physical location and timeframe.

At the point of recognition, we know something has shifted and seek some physiological answers as to 'what' has transpired. There are no words to describe Reiki accurately, no comprehension that can completely define it, no image that encapsulates its beauty, and no song that could ever hope to express the love that we feel when caught up in its embrace. Reiki is literally a catalyst to the experience of touching the Divine... and it is completely overwhelming when you let it into your core awareness. How does your body and brain even begin to describe this seemingly impossible state of being to you in a way that you can consciously understand?

Your body-mind uses a phenomena that has only recently begun to be explored by science—it is the phenomena of synaesthesia. For the longest while, synaesthesia was associated with some form of psychological problem. Children who experienced synaesthesia often ended up being told that what they experienced was 'not real', whilst adults that retained their abilities as a synaesthete, could often end up with psychiatric referrals!

Of course, science (in a very limited understanding of the underlying processes) is now learning that synaesthesia is actually when the brain receives more 'information' that it was expecting and translates the 'extra' chunks of data into a synaesthetic response. I love it when science can make something so utterly enchanting and awe-inspiring sound so... well, boring! Which is why I tend to focus on the experience rather than the explanation of the physiology.

Thus, synaesthesia is a way of your body-mind expressing something that it was not expecting; something that is outside of any usual reference point. Your subconscious brain literally presents you with colours, shapes, sounds, voices, emotions, feelings, tastes, smells, and other sensations, which best describe the 'thing' you are encountering. And by 'thing' I mean 'the entity' that is outside of your usual experience.

With Reiki being a truly and vastly intelligent force, our conscious recognition does not provide a 'static' experience—it is constantly shifting—changing as the interaction takes place. We are whipped into a dialogue of frenetic exchange, where wisdom is instilled within us and you experience Reiki transforming into a reflection of who you are. Your thoughts and those of Reiki interrelate into a rapturous union of expanded awareness where you experience the Divine and the Divine experiences you and all that you are.

In this moment of conscious transference, you desperately try to make sense of things that none of us can ever hope to understand—however, we still do our best; and our best in this instance, is the most profound experience of synaesthesia we can ever know.

It is also in this moment that something very special is occurring, because we are literally translating Divine wisdom through our own perspective and making it physical. We are manifesting the Divine into being 'real'! We remember each nuance and whisper, every hue and spark of joy. And then we take these integral, core experiences into the world and can use them to help others.

From the moment we first experience a connection to the Intelligent Force and the non-physical reality of the Divine that exists within, we are touched by the ability to communicate this (from our own perspective) to other people. When they consciously experience what we present them with, through treatment, consultation, or Orientation, they have the ability to recognise common threads of truth within themselves. When they do this, they shift their focus to their own perspective of Reiki and create a 'direct' connection of their very own.

How we communicate our vReiki Mastery depends on the methods we use... consultation is like a permeating whisper; treatment, a soft and soothing voice; and Orientation a deeply emotional song where the other person joins us in an ever-swelling chorus. Different people respond differently to to the mechanisms of connection; I have known people to experience Reiki when I talk about it, and others become aware during a treatment. Most people, however, first experience their own perspective of Reiki during the Orientation and Calibration process, which we shall look at later in the manual.

As a precursor of what is to come later on your journey, there is a huge difference between another person experiencing your perspective of Reiki (and the other facets of Ki), and knowing their own perspective. Their own, direct connection will always be more profound, unless some form of limiting belief is 'muffling' the interaction.

In many ways, this is how treatment places such an important part in the focus of Reiki Masters of almost all modalities. It is the treatment aspect of our Mastery that enables ourselves and others to transcend the limiting beliefs which stifle our connection to Reiki and the Divine. As we experience treatments from other people, we are immersed on a journey from dis-ease to the ease of wellbeing and health. Once an intent is created for any given treatment, Reiki will literally use the wisdom of the Divine to facilitate a transcendence of whatever the root cause may be. This will, of course, be conducted from the Practitioner's perspective and is why a good rapport is needed with a client!

We shall revisit Practitionership and treatments in the second layer of *The Reiki Revolution Home Experience*. So, let us now turn our attention back to the concept of an 'Intelligent Force' and how Reiki presents so many of the wonderful results that are commonly suggested.

From our very human perspective, the Universe is very complex and seemingly chaotic place. We are often so caught-up in 'overload' that we tend to 'chunk down' to make each day more manageable. This reductive attitude means that we tend to look at surface layer symptoms, rather than deep-level causes. It is why allopathic medicine is separated into parts of human anatomy and physiology, rather than understanding people as whole beings.

As with so many complementary therapies and personal development methods, vReiki treats symptoms as clues to an underlying Core-Self dis-ease. This 'holistic' approach involves treatment of a complete person, rather than their symptoms, however in many holistic practices, there is still a 'chunking down'. Most people understand the holistic approach to take into consideration a person's relationships, diet, home and professional lives, etc. Nonetheless, this is still defining a person in pieces, rather than a whole.

In vReiki Mastery, we focus upon the nature of the Intelligent Force to glean a real appreciation for holism and how it benefits us as people. According to Shinto traditions, the Divine has an over-arcing strategy of ultimate wisdom and it is this which creates life purpose and therefore, life itself. It is the role of Reiki to ensure that the physical Universe is heading towards this ultimate goal, which it does by balancing and harmonising physical reality (the other facets of Ki, as we shall explore later).

The foundation principles of vReiki reflect this philosophy inasmuch as, we are all born in oneness—we are all part of one Universe—yet we experience the illusion of separateness and isolation. To equip us for this lonely journey, we have a life purpose that is uniquely that of the individual. When a person is not living to their life purpose (their passion or raison d'être), they become disconnected from the oneness and eventually become dis-ease at ever-increasing layers of being. When this happens, the physical symptoms are usually at the end of a very long 'backstory' of emotional/psychological/spiritual trauma.

From a human perspective, if we even attempted to understand this vast and convoluted mix of experiences, we would soon lose track, yet Reiki in its powerful knowing, adheres to a simple lore... is a person reflecting their Divine oneness? If not, what needs to change for this to happen? Then Reiki sets about rebalancing and harmonising a person back to oneness, helping them remember that they are truly Divine in nature.

The holism of vReiki is simply that, whatever our treatment type, methodology, or particular perspective, we facilitate one thing: we create a conscious shift of ourselves and others so that we can experience our oneness. To do this, any dis-eases, traumas, fears, and lost-ways are washed away.

This being said, there does need to be a framework, within which the conscious recognition of Reiki takes place... now this could be a loud nightclub or a busy street, but very often the most conducive arena for a conscious sharing of thought between Reiki and people is in a specific type of environment. It is that environment and how we create it that forms the foundations and methods of vReiki. It is these very aspects of Reiki practice that we shall be discovering in this *Home Experience*.

And despite this *Home Experience* being entitled *The Reiki Revolution* and encompassing the arts of vReiki, as we shall see, this is just one aspect of our Mastery. Reiki is merely one facet of Ki, of which there are several more, each with a unique perspective. As we explore this philosophy further, we understand that there is a point where Reiki transitions into another form of Ki in order to create equilibrium. It is at this point of connect that we can focus our Calibration awareness to connect to the other facets of Ki (from a Reiki perspective).

This wondrous ability can be slightly overwhelming at first (not to mention paradoxical, because we shift perspectives with each facet of Ki to sometimes conflicting views or philosophies), yet as we adventure onward on our voyage of discovery, you'll find your ability to perceive from a multitude of perspectives evolves remarkably!

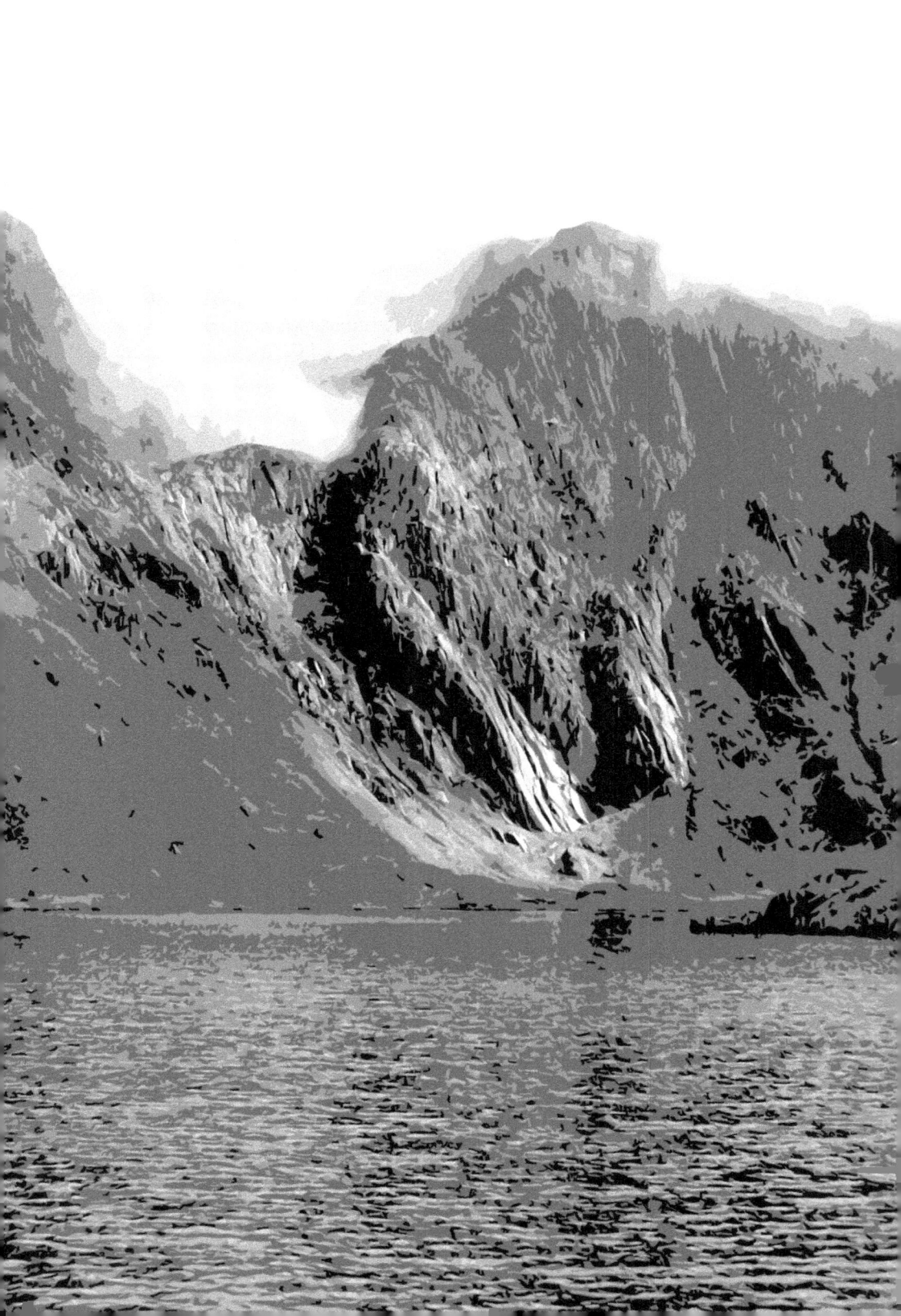

The Ancient Philosophy of Ki

The ancient traditions of the East tell of a mysterious force that creates and encompasses all life. This force is at the foundation of everything in existence, creating dynamics that naturally find balance and harmony, unless hindered by some other factor. The specifics of this force differ from region to region, for example in the Asian subcontinent, this force is known as 'Prana', whilst in China, the term 'Chi' is used.

The traditional sciences of China, such as Feng Shui, observe many different types, or flavours of Chi that are classified by their movement, location, and circumstances, etc. For example, we are all said to inherit Yuan Chi (Conception Chi) from our parents and this regulates the flow of Zheng Chi (Normal Chi) through our bodies. We also have Sheng Chi (Upward Chi), which nurtures life, wealth, and happiness, whilst Sha Chi (Killing Chi) will cause sickness, ill fortune and even death. Additionally, there are individual forms of Chi associated with the elements of water, fire, metal, wood, and earth, whilst the sun and sky also have different variants of Chi.

In Chinese traditions, Chi is so important that if it were to stop flowing through a person for even a fraction of a second, they would be unable to survive the experience. Chi affects our bodies and the way they function, our homes and the lives we lead in them and even our environment including the fortunes of our towns and villages. Chi is the basis of life and death and everything that happens in between.

In the Shinto traditions of Japan, we see another traditional view of this life force, however here it is known as 'Ki'. Whilst the term 'Ki' is not as widely used as its Chinese counterpart (the concept of Chi is widely applied in the practices of Tai Chi, Qigong, and Feng Shui), Ki methodology is found in Reiki modalities, and other Japanese traditions, such as the martial arts of Kiko and Aikido, or the massage therapy of Shiatsu.

In popular culture Chi and Ki become interchangeable although there are distinct differences in the way these forces are seen to operate and function. These variations are in some ways superfluous to all but the enthusiast, however in the study of vReiki, it is essential to understand Ki as being different from other forms of 'life force'. This does not mean that Chi, Ki, Prana and the other forms of life force all coexist. This would invalidate the beliefs behind all of these philosophies (each type of life force is said to be omnipresent and without equal). Yet, when we are discussing a life force in terms of Ki, Chi, etc., we are referring to human perception and traditions rather than the life force itself.

In other words Chi, Ki, and Prana all refer to the same force yet, because we are working with a Japanese tradition in this instance, it is useful to understand how the Japanese perceive this force, as this will have an integral impact to your Mastery of vReiki.

Ki exists in a dynamic and ever-changing balance, where different aspects of Ki have specific tasks to perform in the amazing creation of life. Thus, we can define Ki in many different layers or 'facets' and, by understanding the unique qualities of each facet, so gain a greater understanding of the whole. I believe the act of defining Ki is closer to a sculpting of definition, rather than dividing up and classification of the various facets.

We begin with Shinki, which is the Divine, or the Ki of Kami (Kami is the Shinto concept of the Divine Source). Shinki is essentially non-physical thought; the absolute awareness and vast intelligence of Shinki is so extensive that it knows all things that can be known. The only thing that Shinki does not comprehend is, what it is not to be Shinki. To know everything in oneness and utter connection, presupposes there is no observer to see 'outside' this oneness. Thus, Shinki knows of true love, but has never been kissed for the first time; it understands the joy of birth, yet has never had the experience of being born; it recognises the rose in every turn of petal and prick of thorn, although Shinki has never been moved in awe at the perfume of a rose on a breezy summer's day.

The need to exist outside of itself and to experience separation (and thus reflection) creates life purpose. It is this life purpose that starts an elaborate transformation of Shinki, where layer upon layer of intelligence is folded into an illusion of physicality. This theme of intelligence and physical matter is integral to understanding the Universe within the philosophy of Ki. Shinki creates the illusion of the physical Universe by transforming itself. Conversely, once this deception is complete, it is also all-encompassing and so Shinki cannot affect the realms of physicality. For, whilst Shinki is intelligent beyond all things, it has no actual physical form of its own, so must create a means of bridging the non-physical and physical experience.

For an infinite source to know itself infinitely, an incomprehensible array of experiences need to be consciously explored. These 'moments in time' and the infinite perspectives that perceive these moments soon descend into chaos, so a blueprint is required. This 'master plan' defines everything that has ever happened, is happening, or can ever happen. It details every nuance and how every nuance is created. This is Ishiki; the Ki of Consciousness.

Ishiki has a minute essence of physicality so that it can affect 'reality' in a way that Shinki never can. To attain this sliver of solidity, Ishiki loses a little of Shinki's wisdom. This is fascinating, because not only does it highlight how the balance between wisdom and 'presence in the physical Universe' are so intrinsically linked, it also suggests that there are some elements of Shinki that can never be known in the physical Universe.

As Ishiki maps out an elaborate strategy to fulfil the greater life purpose of all things, further transformations take place as Shinki 'converts' knowledge into physical mass. Wrapping itself into the illusion of our solid world, Shinki creates the Ki of Blood; Kekki, which is the strongest and most physically powerful of all Ki. Kekki is the ability to nourish and grow; it is the raw material from which all physical matter developed. If we imagine a huge city fashioned from buildings made of brick, Kekki is the clay that creates that brick. Wherever there is group interaction, bonding between people and social connection, we find Kekki, as these are the elements of life that create it. Yet Kekki, despite its physical potency, cannot exist without something to nourish and a place to be, so other facets of Ki were formed to continue the processes of life.

Shioke is the Ki of Salt and behaves as a receptacle for Kekki, merging with it, but preserving the individual characteristics of both. If Kekki is seen as the clay, Shioke can be perceived as the bricks derived from it; the building blocks integral to all life. It is said that the physical body is actually formed from these two aspects of Ki, moulded from their synthesis in order to fulfil the life purpose of Shinki. Indeed, Shioke mirrors this life purpose (according to Ishiki), for it is created whenever we discover an objective or reason for living. Whilst we are striving and moving towards our goals, Shioke is with us enabling our reflection of the Divine. Shioke is credited with the life span of our cells and our physical bodies, for we only need live as long as we choose to in order to accomplish our dreams; once we have done what we came to do, we no longer need to be here and so Shioke enables our departure from life as well as our appearance into it.

Mizuke, the Ki of Water, is the catalyst for communication and enables the combination of Kekki and Shioke to form complex structures. Mizuke is expansion, reproduction and growth. In this trinity of Ki facets it continually strives to further itself and to produce a greater scale of life and physical being. The tenacity of Mizuke is echoed in life, forming the basis of our emotions, sexuality and body awareness. We create Mizuke through communication with each other and in the development of intimate relationships.

Wherever there is expansion, there must also be restraint for, if these three aspects of Ki could endlessly grow, there would merely be a huge mass of physical matter without boundary or division. So in limitation we discover the diversity of Kuki, the Ki of Air.

Kuki is the initiator of boundaries that regulate the growth of Kekki, Shioke, and Mizuke. It is these borders that facilitate the concepts of individuality and separateness as they mask our connection to each other and with all things. Kuki is the facet of Ki that offers the illusion of you, me and them, the table, the chair and so on. Kuki provides us with our awareness and basic perception; it is consciousness and how we perceive the world around us.

In separation Kuki also binds us by instilling within each of us a mutual rhythm, a common goal. It is this that drives and motivates us, making us individuals yet causing us to seek connection with others through our relationships, families, cultural groups, communities and so on. It is with our interactions, our self-recognition and the shaping of our lives that Kuki is created.

As we find connection with each other and escape our isolation, we discover love, the embodiment of the Ki of Thunder, Denki. Denki is at the root of all human experience, it nurtures acceptance although it also has associations with cleansing as it teaches us through fear of loss and heartache. The Ki of Thunder is like the storm that cuts through stagnation and stillness, provoking movement and a purging of the things we no longer require. It is through the lessons of Denki and the love it makes possible that we strive for our life purpose and discover the origins of our being here. By following our path and discovering both love and loss on our way, we learn how to experience empathy and compassion: qualities that create Denki.

As each individual becomes aware of their uniqueness and meaning, they meet others and form loving connections; they develop social groups, cultural communities, large populations and so forth. With people experiencing their own private motivations and priorities we observe the formation of complex dynamics, which need to be supported, directed, and to a certain extent governed. It is in this function that Jiki is created and the Ki of Magnetism guides us both individually and at the level of group consciousness.

Jiki is charismatic, symbolising beauty and harmony in all things. Whenever groups work together to produce or uncover something good, it is Jiki that channels their effort and brings it to fruition. Jiki oversees our awareness on the larger scale in relation to our society, faith, race and species; leading us onwards, we are drawn together by its magnetism in order to find our unique cultural routes to truth and beauty.

It is Jiki that offers awareness to the other facets of Ki discussed so far, thus presenting them with the ability to act together for the unified good of all things. This particular layer of Ki creates a magnetic attraction amongst the other layers, bringing them closer and managing the overall progression.

Which leads us to the mysterious Tsuki; the Ki of the Moon. Here the underlying dynamics of the physical world are experienced at a level of consciousness. If each aspect of Ishiki exists in potential, the Tsuki equivalent would be the complete understanding of this aspect as it exists in the physical world. For example, if the potential for an entire ocean exists in the plan of Ishiki, the memory of swimming in that ocean would be the domain of Tsuki. For Tsuki exists wherever physical beings create conscious thought and therefore strive to realise the life purpose of Shinki.

It is interesting to note that when we experience the synaesthesia created by our interaction with Reiki, it is Tsuki that symbolises those experiences. We could view this dynamic as a mirror, where Reiki is the reflective surface, Ishiki the source and Tsuki the reflection. Therefore, Tsuki acts as the reward for everything that has gone before; the ultimate goal of conscious experience and the precursor to a return to Shinki, because Tsuki is also the facet of Ki that recognises itself as Shinki. Tsuki, for all its mysteries and enigma is actually where we lift the veil of illusion and discover ourselves as the Divine. Tsuki is the memory of our oneness and a call home to where the loneliness and separation of the physical world is no more.

This is also where a strange side effect of existence occurs, for when we approach Tsuki, we have had plenty of time to develop an ego-self, through the actions of Kuki, Denki, and Jiki. This ego recognises the illusion of its own existence and fights to deny the reality of oneness—for oneness means losing self-definition and to the ego, this is an absolutely terrifying prospect. What is it like not to be me? What happens when my consciousness is no more? And so on. Hence, it is with Tsuki that both life and death meet in a crucible of experience, both joyous and painful to behold.

This leads us to the final facet of Ki and perhaps the best known: Reiki, or the Ki of the Soul. Reiki is a bridge between the pure wisdom of Shinki and the material nature of the other facets of Ki. Reiki is the organiser and equalising force of life that accomplishes its aim by balancing all facets of 'physically-orientated' Ki. In creating equilibrium in-line with the blueprint of Ishiki, Reiki helps us fulfil life purpose and rediscover oneness with all things. With a highly intelligent nature, Reiki understands the physical being in a way that Shinki cannot and hence, acts as representative of the Divine in our physical world.

It is believed that, when in balance, the facets of Ki create perfection of all things, yet if these different layers of Ki fall out of alignment, we soon see the development of dis-ease, which filters down through each aspect of Ki, from Jiki to Kekki. When one loses sight of life purpose, it leads to mental and emotional unrest. Social and cultural issues soon arise from this discordance and we feel cut off, abandoned and alone. When this happens we try to readdress the imbalance by focusing on physical solutions, relying on addiction and codependence to compensate; this in turn, leads to physical disease.

Reiki rebalances all the aspects of Ki by bridging the gap between physical and spiritual by using the knowledge of Shinki to bring the physical aspects of Ki back into alignment. By re-establishing balance, Reiki creates oneness on all levels and develops a path for us to define our own, personal relationship with the Shinki—our oneness with/as the Divine.

This concept may seem a little difficult to translate into everyday life—especially in early 21st Century Western Culture! However, the practicalities are that we can experience an interaction with Reiki at all levels of our being. This in turn creates specific results such as physical healing, success and accomplishment, creating emotional balance, positive thinking, harmonising relationships, and evolving spiritual enlightenment. By using a range of techniques, we can train ourselves to focus on the areas of our lives that we wish to 'make better' and shift Reiki into consciousness at this point of our being or life.

We can view the force of Reiki as we would that of electricity. Reiki is the power to create some form of change within a person or situation, yet we need to develop a conscious interaction with Reiki at that specific point. So, we need to add different tools and techniques to give the Reiki something to 'power'. With electricity, we provide something for it to power such as a TV set, CD player, light bulb, heater, etc. By itself, electricity just 'is'. However, when directed through electronic equipment, we can use it to create a myriad array of effects and tailor those effects to provide us with an endless amount of uses.

It is valuable to note at this juncture that many people confuse the concept of Reiki (force) with Reiki therapies and practices. The main instance of this is when Usui Reiki is referred to as simply 'Reiki'. This would be the equivalent of calling a TV, 'electricity'! Imagine a world where every electronic device was simply named 'electricity' and you can see how all kinds of misunderstandings would arise. Thus, it is always important to distinguish between the force of Reiki and the methodology we are working with (in this case, vReiki).

Techniques and tools construct the framework of the therapy that we use and the Reiki powers those techniques. This means that interacting with Reiki at certain areas of focus creates a change of some variety. Usually in Reiki modalities, we are encouraged to divide up our needs into specific 'symptoms'; such as to heal an injured knee, or solving a problem that is affecting somebody's emotional wellbeing. Nonetheless, the Intelligent Force will always exist in the perspective of holism. Reiki does not flow or travel or appear somewhere where it was not before, it is infinite and therefore exists at all points of the Universe in an incomprehensible array of potential states of being... it is us that experience the sense of flow through synaesthesia and natural physiology responses to the changes Reiki creates.

An excellent way of understanding how Reiki can be used is to imagine the dynamics of our Universe. Take a moment to imagine what is happening in your body, from the flow of blood through your arteries and veins, the beat of your heart, the impulses that travel through your nerves, the chemicals that act and react with your cells, the thoughts in your head and the movement of your muscles. Each of these interactions creates a dynamic and these dynamics affect each other to form complex layers of dynamics, all working towards a common goal. Everything we do in our life is based on the dynamics that are within us and around us.

Each time we interact with another person, or work through a situation, we are forming new dynamics that once again build into systemic, dynamic structures. Add to this all living things, our weather, our environment, the oceans and the movement of our planet, the sun, moon and stars and before long we begin to see that our Universe is a place of unimaginable complexity and beauty. As the Universe exists around us and within us, we are guiding it and are guided by it. Yet every action and move we make will take place in in a way that is conducive to some systems and negates others. If we increase the level of beneficial dynamics and eradicate those that sabotage us, life is easy and joyful, but if we negate our supportive systems of dynamics and encourage contractive systems, we often encounter challenges.

So how do we know what are the best moves to make in order to maintain wellbeing? How do we change the dynamics that are not conducive to our wellbeing and happiness? How do we choose the best areas to focus upon, or what actions to take for our greater good? Well, according to Japanese tradition, Shinki, the Divine Ki knows every single dynamic and understands the perfection of it all. This plan, in the form of Ishiki, can be facilitated through Reiki in order to guide us through all the chaos and complexity.

Thus, acting as a bridge between perfect understanding and the other facets of Ki that in turn influence everything from physical growth to social communication, Reiki is the catalyst that can heal relationships or boost the healing agents in the bloodstream. It can nurture the correction of chemical imbalance or assist large groups of people working towards a common goal. (Remember, this is all completed by reintroducing oneness and life purpose.)

When we understand this about Reiki, we see that the Ki of the Soul refers not to an individual soul, but to the soul of all things; the journey that we all must make to achieve our Divine oneness. It is the very essence of who we are and also everything that we do. By consciously 'noticing' the effects of Reiki, we are guided by its wisdom and learn from its teachings, revelling within its beauty and exploring how to adapt our own methodology to closely reflect that of Reiki. With every experience of Reiki, we initiate a process that ensures we holistically enrich our lives in more ways than we can imagine!

Ki and a Modern Reality

In our 21st Century world, the ancient Japanese concept of Ki may seem somewhat strange, tending to be incongruous with our perception of how 'things' work in our physical reality. Yet, even as early as the 1920's, scientists have known that our physical realm is not as we believe it to be.

We perceive our world through our senses, understanding that because we touch something it is real; that seeing is believing. However, the world that we can sense so well and that appears to be so real, is actually created entirely of energy, a force that is only detectable to a certain extent. Our senses have evolved through adaptation, mainly to ensure the survival of our physical bodies and are intensively focused upon this goal. Yet there is so much beyond the reach of our senses that in modern society we have become highly sceptical of. The arrogance of humankind is to believe that we each have a good grasp of 'reality' and what the 'real world' is like. In actuality, all we can truly know is our own version of reality!

From a scientific perspective, even the most sophisticated sensory machines can only detect a minute fraction of the energy, from which all is created, to a certain level of detail. What lies beyond the boundaries of our sensing equipment is the realm of mathematical theory and those who use their synaesthete abilities to sense what exists outside the range of average perception—and indeed even in these incidences, we can only speculate and hypothesise to the actual reality of what is experienced.

A philosophical debate regarding human experience could go on a long time (and has!), however I will leave this particular tangent by offering an example... It was not that long ago that people in the Western world believed it to be okay to torture and burn others for witchcraft (a nebulous term that often meant a person possessed a cat, warts, and bottles of herbs in there kitchen!). They were not 'playing' at burning witches—this practice was perfectly legal at the time—it was the reality of many of our ancestors. They totally believed they understood how the world worked and what must be done to save these people's souls (and their own). Looking back we may wince when we think of the atrocities that transpired, yet we are equally naive to the infinite wisdom of actual reality and, furthermore, I doubt any human—individual or community—will ever truly know what 'it' is all about! We can merely do the best with the tools (and perspective) that we have at any given moment.

When we encounter something that is bigger or more complex than we can comprehend, we have been taught to 'chunk down' into smaller parts, until we can grasp all the 'little bits', before putting them back together. Whilst this method works very well for mathematical equations or technological equipment, encounters that are essentially creative or spiritual in nature cannot be understood using this philosophy.

People whose primary thinking modality is from their left-hand brain are most likely to break the whole into little pieces with everything they don't understand. If those little pieces still do not make any sense, most will dismiss the 'whole' as incomprehensible, or nonsense.

When we encounter a spiritual or creative practice, the right-hand brain approach is to maintain wholeness as much as possible, whilst 'sculpting' definition into a 'memorable form'.

Unfortunately, decades of this left-brain approach to holistic medicine and spiritual, including Reiki practices, means that we have ended up with a conglomeration of bits and bobs. Chunks, bolted together into a clunky, inflexible tangle of methods. Many are skeptical about the validity of Reiki therapies, others are dogmatic and rigid in their beliefs. Reiki Mastery is not seen as a beautifully defined and nuanced sculpture, but as a range of 'do this and do thats', which are 'right' or 'wrong'.

The Mastery of vReiki is based upon taking an ancient philosophy and, rather than breaking into smaller bits, we redefine these beliefs for a modern perspective. This repositioning in the way we understand Reiki means that we develop a much greater level of fluidity and individuality in our practices. Thus, vReiki is about your Reiki, instead of Reiki practices that you must conform to.

Our sculpting approach, when applied to the philosophy of Reiki, enables us to comprehend a seamless and extremely potent reality where we can be human, with all the smiles, tears, faults, and foibles, yet remain in constant oneness with the Divine. I understand this to be a perspective of further dimensions that expands the usual narrow shaft of consciousness we are used to, therefore achieving greater personal truth within, and less dogma without.

This is something you may experience for yourself over the next few months, because as we explore the unlimited perspective of Ki and our experience of the Divine, and compare this to the traditional techniques of Reiki Mastery (as they are usually taught), you'll see how one appears very 'mechanical' next to the other. This is not a 'bad' thing, it is simply a different thing... and different things please different people!

On of the most basic areas of Reiki experience that we address right here, at the beginning of the path, is that of flow. The term 'flow' is a wonderful expression of emotion and human experience. When we are in 'flow', we achieve unimaginable wonders. We know that 'going with the flow' offers an easy road ahead and that the sensation of flowing is really magical. Although, when it comes to any modality of Reiki Mastery, the concept of 'flow' actually sabotages us.

Flow is one of the most common pieces of feedback that people offer when interacting with Reiki. We talk about feeling the flow down our arms or through our body. We visualise showers of light travelling down, through the top of the head and onwards, filtering into every part of the body. I have not met a single Reiki Master of any modality that does not speak in terms of flow and even I was trained to speak that way—and did for many years!

Yet all is not as we believe it to be. For flow is our sensation, not Reiki. To truly interact with Reiki, there is a need to transcend the human perception that binds us and 'speak the language of Reiki'.

Energy is infinite, the concept of flow limits this—we flow, not Reiki. In other words Reiki is all powerful and all wise, yet over time, we experience a strengthening of power and wisdom, not because Reiki has become stronger or wiser, but due to our experience of Reiki becoming more integral to our Core-Self.

If Reiki flows down the arm, what exists at the hand, when the flow of Reiki reaches the elbow? Are we saying Reiki does not exist at the hand at this point in time? I believe that Reiki exists at all points of our being at all times—whether we are aware of this consciously is another matter! Thus it is we that flow through time and consciousness to experience Reiki, rather than Reiki being non-existent (therefore limited) at certain points of the physical world, at certain times.

The sensation of flow that many experience during treatment or practice is more a result of our nervous system and the impulses firing in the neurones, than the flow of Reiki. In other words as each neurone fires with the recognition of Reiki, we translate this as a flow. In turn this is often misinterpreted as a flow of energy, rather than our nervous system communicating in a chain-like method.

Our experience is of flow, not Reiki. Reiki simply 'is'. This is a concept that most struggle with, many resist, and few master. Yet if you can master the concept of Reiki existing in every aspect of the Universe, thus transcending the reductive notion of flow, you will discover the context of your physical body within infinity. To do so, shifts your perspective from the rigidly defined ego-self you have been confined to, and opens your perception to the limitless potential you truly are.

To fully know the Divine, we need to step so far into our (non-physical) Shinki potential that we cannot remain physical beings. However, we can shift into a limitless Reiki perspective and experience Ishiki. This enables us to touch the Divine, without losing our connection to physicality. We shall be learning how to achieve this awe-inspiring state of being at the Master degree of *The Reiki Revolution Home Experience*.

In physicality, we are bound by our human form and viewpoint. Nonetheless, we can ingress into the very core of our being and experience Reiki in a truly infinite way. In a Viridian (v) perspective, this translates to a powerful change in perspective, where we glimpse the transpersonal, non-human perception that drives us. I refer to this as 'Plexi'. Our Plexible friends will be joining us later, but for now let us investigate an area where tradition is utterly indispensable...

You'll notice that I use the term 'Ki', never 'Kis'. I write about 'facets of Ki', not 'various Kis'. And there is always a sense that we are interacting with a defined area that extends into a whole entity of oneness, rather than autonomous, or separate pieces. There is a very good reason for this. The Eastern traditions we use as a foundation respect and truly appreciate 'oneness', and how all things in existence strive for wholeness. We are all the Divine, not in some broken and fragmented way, but in a perfectly sculpted unity of one. Every facet of the Divine is precious and is as vital as any other.

In modern society we have been taught a very reductive attitude to life... the aforementioned 'chunking' seems omnipresent, and whilst breaking a complex task in bits, or a book into chapters may help us comprehend the whole, in spiritual terms it simply diminishes our potential and joy in staggering ways. The physical world and the etheric are based on different laws/lores (as the complexity of human life increases we are finding a shift to a more 'etheric logic' of sculpting is also vital in the physical world!).

When we commit our lives and legacy to truly touching the Divine, we need to 'rewrite the internal script' or 'reprogram our software' to ensure that we attain the necessary perspective of an unlimited view. The traditional approach to Ki honours this oneness with the expression of one 'Ki' and not 'Kis'. In modern spirituality we forget this and use term 'energies'. Did you feel me shudder there? Even the need to write the word once (and I will not write it again!) causes a physical aversion in my being, because I have placed such importance on not using the word.

I used to use this term as frequently as any other Reiki Master or Energy Therapist, but when I began to grasp how detrimental it was to my spiritual wellbeing, I set about purging it from my vocabulary. Once rid of the offending word, I spent years with the deeply engrained concept of 'energy' as one force, with infinite perspectives/facets, and this has taught me how truly toxic the aforementioned plural is.

Now, I understand what people are referring to when they chunk energy. I know what 'Earth Energy' is, when compared to 'my energy' or 'your energy'. Yes, I am almost in the foetal position now! Of course I get the gist of what they are referring to, however every time we express the concept of energy as being a fragmented array of different 'things' we corrupt the very thing that makes it more than our human perspective... its oneness. The 'e-word' that I deplore with such fervour, I believe, is the refined sugar of the spiritual word. It commits the ethereal equivalent of rotting our teeth, causing obesity, and literally making addicts out of us with its saucy wiles.

I hardly ever present absolutes in my teachings, because I cherish other people's perspectives, and it is because of that respect that I have so much disgust for what seems to be such an inoffensive word.

One aspect of vReiki (and the other therapies I have originated) which is absolutely essential to achieving the full potential of experience and Mastery, is that the 'e*******' word is irrevocably exorcised from your vocabulary. And before you sit wide-eyed and wondering why the tirade; think about 'a complete body detox with doughnuts'—one negates the other, so they compete until one gets the upper hand... a healthier body or a trip to Krispy Kreme's (or Timmy's for my Canadian readers!).

Now ask yourself why should the task of 'not using that word' create such resistance. If you have ever done a complete body detox, you will probably understand the cravings... well, from experience, the best way I equate the perniciousness of that word is with those cravings for sugary foods when starved of them. If you're not a fan of sugar (or complete body cleanses), think about alcohol, cigarettes, TV, obsessive behaviour, or anything that you, personally feel compelled to do, even though you know it is not conducive to your wellbeing.

Our habitual need to divide up the most powerful spiritual concept (and the words we label the resulting carnage as) is an exercise in control. To transcend the control the concept behind the word has upon us, the word itself needs to be eradicated. This will, I assure you, make perfect sense a little ways along the path, which is why we need to explore the way we 'frame' certain concepts in our Mastery, so early on in this *Home Experience*.

So, now that we have had a moment's pause for a Glazed Chocolate Cream (or a Double Double with Tim Bits), let us merrily return to our beautifully formed singular concept of energy!

Energy creates the foundation for all things. It is all around us and within us and at every single place in the Universe. It simply 'is'. Most of the time this energy exists as non-physical potential, although it also exists as certain forms of physical energy (light, electricity, gravity, etc.), or it 'interacts' into solid matter. Energy is described in scientific terms as 'force' or the 'power to achieve some result' and is available in many forms, be these physical, subtle or potential. The philosophy of Ki is applied to facets of energy that are recognised from particular viewpoints; e.g. the Shinto perspective, etc. Just as a diamond has many facets, Ki is a facet of energy and it is energy.

Ki is often referred to as 'subtle energy', which means it is beyond the usual scope of human sensory perception (and very often outside the range of scientific sensing equipment also... mainly because these machines are based on the human perspective and thus, limited by it).

Interestingly enough, when a scientist called John Zimmerman created a sensory device that could detect vibrations of energy well below the usual limit, he discovered that every organ of the body actually vibrates at a very low frequency. When he recorded the vibration rate of an Usui Reiki Master's hands, he found the range of frequencies detected matched those of the body and continued to an even higher range. It was therefore surmised that by working with the experience of Ki, we could create vibrations that match those of a 'conducive healing environment'. So if a broken bone vibrates at 7Hz when it is healing, a Reiki Master's hands vibrating at 7Hz will speed the process up, and so on (it is debatable whether the 7Hz is actually Reiki, the Practitioner's own resonance, or the client's resonance when interacting with Reiki!).

The higher range of frequencies that are produced in Reiki treatments are said to work on emotional and mental layers of the self, thus anything over 20Hz is firmly in the realms of healing emotional trauma and mental illness. We can even measure the vibrations of energy that work with spiritual enlightenment and phenomena such as astral travel and ESP.

Since Zimmerman's discoveries in the 1980's, his work has been well quoted and used, not only in the circles of Reiki practice, but also in a wide range of metaphysical works that have focused on healing. The much larger body of research into Quantum Physics, which is the study of very small particles and the energy contained within them, has had even greater value to the esoteric community and is often quoted as proof of subtle energy.

In actuality this does not cause any harm, as much of the information, both scientific and esoteric, is theoretical anyway. However, while scientists devise experiments to (dis)prove their theories and progress in their field, most Reiki modality Practitioners and Teachers tend to let science hold them back. By quoting the findings of Zimmerman, et al, and not getting to grips with the concepts and terminology used, I've seen many people quote verbatim and rarely delve any deeper.

In recent years, the way we interact with Ki (and other perspectives of life force) has changed and evolved, initiating an exciting new age in energy medicine. These changes have so far been limited to other forms of therapy or self-development tools, however with vReiki, the most advanced methodologies have been applied to the ancient techniques and views; so creating a very different breed of Reiki modality.

The Universe is expanding. It is always changing and developing and, as an intrinsic part of the Universe, we undergo those changes also. In the last few years, massive changes in the

Universe meant that the way we experience Reiki practices and other energy medicine forms would not be as effective as before. These changes are known as an 'energy-shift'. These shifts are common with at least 2–3 happening every month. Most affect us only minimally, but one shift in May 2005 was integral to our being and heralded an era that is very different to what has gone before.

The major difference is the method of interaction with Reiki as opposed to changes in the Intelligent Force itself. In traditional (and indeed modern) views, a person becomes unwell and the 'administering of Reiki' can help them to heal; a person holds on to trauma, Reiki can help them release this and gradually rise above their trauma; and so on. We could view this as a journey or pathway from dis-ease to health or from trauma to enlightenment. Since the shift of 2005, the intent of moving along a path no longer creates results in the same way as pre-shift. As our conscious experience of time moves away from the shift, the more we see the diminishing success in treatment outcomes.

Of course, with any Universal change, we adapt and find our own way to modify our interactions (not only with Reiki, but with all things). The strategies of vReiki simply make the transition processes that are taking place, quicker, smother, and more potent that when evolving by default. In other regions of the *Home Experience*, we shall explore the concept of energy-shifts and how they have, not only irrevocably reshaped our journey of Mastery, but also initiated the Reiki Revolution.

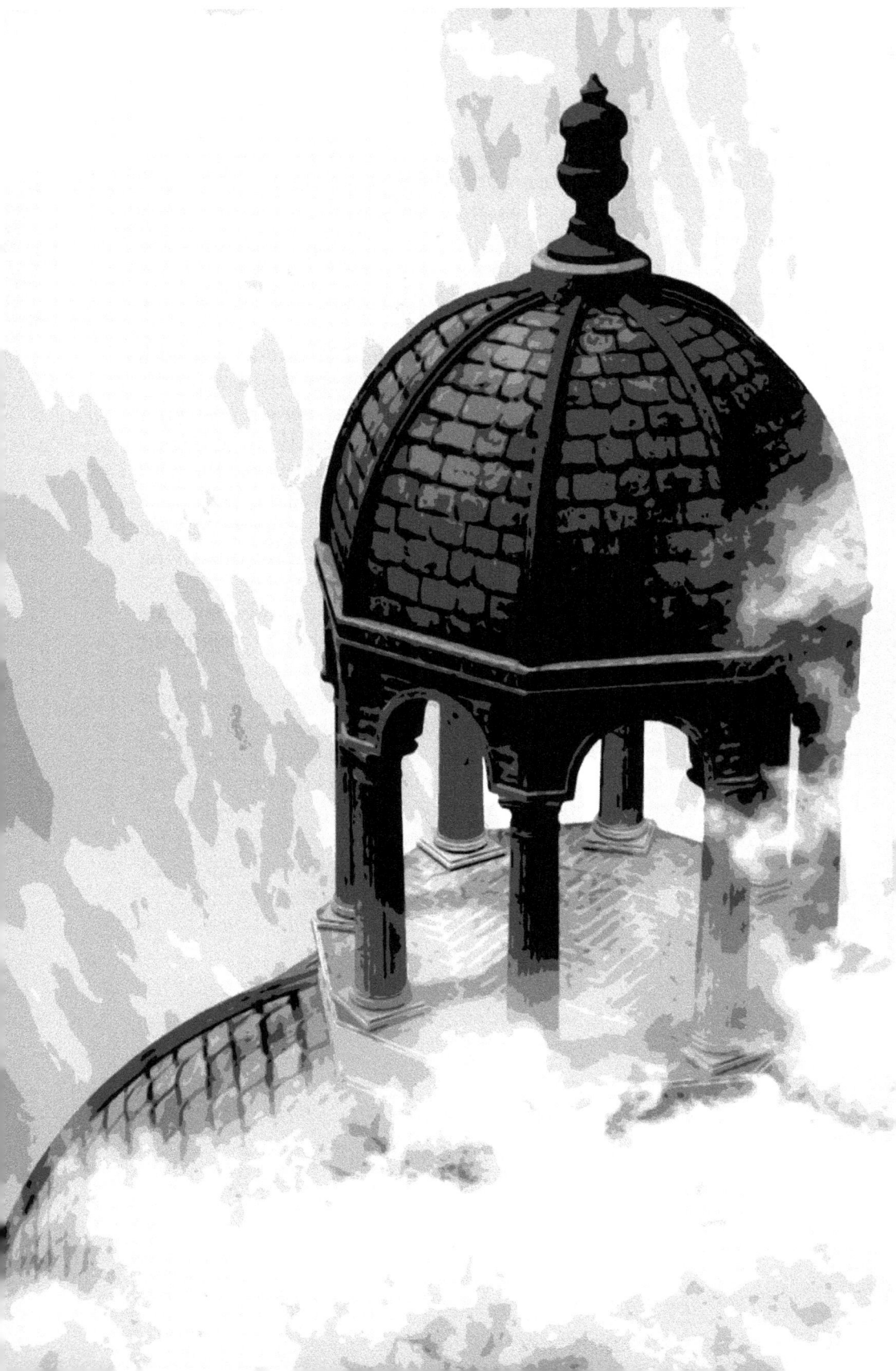

The Temple

The History and Development of Usui Reiki

The most common form of therapy that uses Reiki is known as Usui Reiki Ryoho, often abbreviated to Usui Reiki. As we have already seen, the term 'Reiki' was used to describe a facet of Ki that had been a part of Shintoism for thousands of years, yet it was made popular when used by a man named Mikao Usui who was born in the village of Yago in the Yamagata district of Gifu prefecture, Japan, on August 15, 1865.

Much has been said about Usui and his life but very little can be substantiated. He has been described as a Christian Missionary who travelled the world on a quest to explain the healing powers of Christ. Others say that he was raised in a Tendai Buddhist Monastery and during this time he was exposed to many different forms of Ki using techniques, such as Kiko and a martial art known as Yagyu Ryu. The latter is the more likely of the two scenarios as it is known that much of Usui's history was 'rewritten' to make it more palatable to a largely Christian, Western society.

What is known about Usui is that he was married with two children and, before originating his Reiki techniques, he had been left with many debts after a failed business venture. As a man, he appears to have been driven by a profound need to discover a greater meaning to life and a deep fascination with spirituality. He lived in a period of great flux when Japan had been made to open its borders to the world and a rapid phase of transition took place.

As Japan was transformed from a feudal society to an industrialised nation, there was a real desire to embrace new ideas and cultures while retaining the old beliefs and traditions.

Usui Reiki was born of this synthesis of the old and the new. Usui took advantage of this flood of new information as he supplemented his experience with the ancient Buddhist Ki practices, with knowledge of Western Medicine, mystic arts such as numerology and astrology as well as the development of psychic abilities.

Whilst on a retreat at Mount Kurama (a holy mountain near Kyoto, the former capital of Japan), Mikao Usui entered upon a 21-day meditation and fast called 'The Lotus Repentance', which is derived from Tendai Buddhism. According to Usui's memorial stone, he experienced a 'satori' that led to the development of his Reiki practice. A satori is a brief moment of enlightenment or glimpse of oneness and the profound wisdom that could be compared to that of an epiphany. During his satori, Usui was totally enveloped by a light or force that he later referred to as Reiki.

After this life-changing experience, Usui set about developing a way to use this powerful life force for creating satori. Referring to his Kiko training, Usui used the graceful movements of this ancient practice to entrain, focus and alter his interactions with Reiki to his intent. Developing processes that could be used for healing the self and others, practices of deep meditation and reflection and also methods for increasing one's spiritual and physical connection to the Intelligent Force. Usui's real masterpiece was in the creation of the attunement or energy lesson that enabled him to interact with Reiki in such a way that others could perceive it and interact with it as he had done.

The technique he created, known as the Reiju Empowerment, offered a permanent connection to Reiki that would never leave a student and could be used with the techniques Usui created to offer great ability. Using Reiju, Usui 'empowered' nearly 2000 students to Reiki, supplementing their learning with the techniques derived from Kiko and spiritual teachings.

Originally entitled 'teate' (pronounced tee-ah-tay), meaning 'hand healing' or 'hand application', the Usui system underwent many changes from its earliest inception. The addition of tools that enabled practitioners to change the way Reiki behaves and the addition of various healing methods created a very different practice to the original form Usui originated.

Mikao Usui died on March 9th, 1926: it is said that he succumbed to a stroke whilst teaching his method to a group of Usui Reiki One students. According to Usui's Memorial stone, he was a very well known and popular healer, who taught a large number of students all over Japan, including 17 people trained to Master level.

Although Usui Reiki is generally perceived in the West as a healing system, the original focus of Usui Reiki methodology was the personal benefits that are experienced through the system. As a self-development practice, Usui Reiki was aimed at knowing one's true purpose in life, discovering contentment, healing the self, finding a spiritual path and ultimately achieving satori. The emphasis upon Usui Reiki as a healing method was instigated by one of Usui's students; a man named Dr. Chujiro Hayashi.

Hayashi came from a medical and military background and strived to instil a greater degree of structure to the Usui system. Keeping detailed records of every person he treated, Hayashi created a training handbook that gave prescriptive hand positions to treat specific diseases. Hayashi used this as a way of enabling students to learn the advanced scanning and intuitive techniques while using the standard hand positions as a supporting methodology.

Hayashi is also responsible for developing an attunement process of greater complexity, which used cerebral triggers (sometimes known as the 'Reiki Symbols'). He taught students over a fixed number of days, involving a rigid framework that was vastly removed from the informal methods employed by Usui. In view of these major changes, Hayashi founded his own society in 1931 called Hayashi Reiki Kenyu-kai, respecting his master's training by altering the name in order to maintain the integrity of the Usui system.

One of the patients that visited Hayashi's clinic was Hawayo Takata who, despite her misgivings and scepticism regarding Reiki practice, was treated for various diseases. Born in 1900 on the island of Kauai, Hawaii, Mrs Takata was so impressed by her recovery when treated with Reiki therapy that she became the first person not born in Japan to be trained to Master level.

Upon completion of her training in 1938, Mrs Takata was given permission by Hayashi to teach Reiki practices in the West. This she did, opting to train students in the United States at a time, after the Second World War, when memories of Pearl Harbour were still fresh in people's minds and anything 'Japanese' was deeply mistrusted.

Since that time, the world has evolved in many ways and we are much more open to the concepts of Ki/Chi and the methodology of Eastern Arts. During Mrs Takata's time however, things would have seemed very alien to her students and so the Usui Reiki Mastery training was altered once again with even shorter workshops, simplified hand positions and a completely modified history. It was this factor, which introduced the idea of Usui as a Christian Missionary.

During the period from 1970 to her death in 1980, Mrs Takata taught 22 people to the degree of Usui Reiki Master and thus initiated the spread of Usui Reiki practice to countries all over the world including Japan, where the practice of Usui Reiki was believed to have died out except for a few isolated Usui Reiki groups. In the 1990's when Western Reiki Masters moved to Japan, they were able to share knowledge with these rare Usui practitioners and thus rediscovered the origins of Reiki practice.

It is estimated that there are now millions of people in the world who have trained to use Reiki practices of one form or another. Due to the ever changing and developing nature of the Reiki practices, including several hundred different 'modalities' of Reiki practice now in existence, there is often heated debate as to which is the 'right' and 'wrong' way to practise.

Although the practice of Usui Reiki is now often bound in a realm of dogma, social politics and personal power struggles, the force behind it all, Reiki, remains a beautiful and powerful intelligence that can change lives in unimaginable ways. However, the manner in which this is done is often so wrapped up in egocentricities that it takes a lot of faith to see past the other 'stuff', thus causing many to dismiss Reiki practitioners as arrogant and the practice as a means to gratify the ego.

In the past few years things have started to change. Various members of the Reiki practice community are so upset at seeing their beloved therapy fought over and tarnished that new versions of the original system have started to arise. Some of these are close to the original principles of Mikao Usui, while other modalities use very different methodologies from Usui-style therapy.

vReiki is one of these new forms of practice and was created specifically to redefine Reiki practice for a very different world to the one that Usui lived in. In the very same way Mikao Usui, using a fusion of old and new techniques, originated that Reiki practice, so vReiki ventures right back to the origins of the Shinto philosophies surrounding Ki and an array of completely new methods for the 'Viridian Age'.

Understanding why this is so important is vital to the vReiki Master, because when we recreate traditional practices, they may be insufficient to meet the needs of a modern lifestyle. For instance, The handbook of Dr Hayashi mentions treatments for disease that one would hardly ever encounter in the 21st Century and several hand positions that would be highly inappropriate in a contemporary treatment environment! Usui Reiki in all its adaptations was originated to cater to client's needs at the time and without reworking to envelop the complexity of our lives now, it simply cannot achieve the results we need.

This is a point that, again, is highly refuted by many Usui Reiki Masters, yet if we view the challenges we take into consideration developments such as the Internet, Social Media and the way we communicate, this has literally changed the way many people think and the therapy needs to reflect this. Hold on a minute... but surely Reiki is intelligent enough to adapt to modern needs? Yes, the intelligent Ki of the Soul is, as you would expect, fully conversant with human lifestyles now and into the future, however it is the way we interact with Reiki that gives potency to the treatment in our physical Universe. Interactions at a more expanded layer of consciousness create more effective treatments.

So, on this journey, we shall begin with the foundations of traditional Reiki methods, created by Usui, Hayashi, Takata and others. We then continue onwards to the evolution of vReiki and our Viridian Age philosophy of Reiki. This journey will be varied and offer many different perspectives; some of which you may resonate with, others not so much. Either way, they are presented to you so that you can glean an idea of just how varied Reiki Mastery is and what you can make of it on your own, unique terms.

Before we head off for an exploration of some more recent developments to Reiki practices, let us examine one of the cornerstones of Usui Reiki Mastery. In his teachings, Mikao Usui used the poetry of Japan's Meiji Emperor to emphasize the spiritual nature of using the Ki of the Soul. From the many poems, he devised a set of principles that can used to help Usui Reiki Mastery on a daily basis. The value of these principles is still apparent as the observation of each precept creates a mantra to guide us when developing an initial connection to Reiki.

The principles are not seen as rules, but as guidelines that can recalled at times of need and form part of routine that will assist your ability to entrain to the Usui perspective of Reiki.

Just for today...

...Do not anger

...Do not worry

...Be thankful

...Endeavour in work

...Nurture dharma for your teachers

...Be kind to all living things

Anger: The first two principles are interesting, because in Eastern philosophy that are no 'good' or 'bad' emotions—all emotions are neutral, it is the repression or exaggeration of emotions that cause dis-ease. Particularly in Western society, we are taught to stifle anger and seek our joy. Yet the more we bottle up anger, the more likely it is to explode from us in the future. Repression of anger can also make us unwell, causing various diseases and emotional traumas. We should acknowledge our anger by letting it focus us, propel us forward and then just let it go.

Worry: In Eastern medicine, worry is often referred to as 'pensiveness' and again is not viewed as a 'bad' emotion. The things we worry about are rarely the things that hurt us—it's what we don't see coming that knocks us off our feet. When we fixate on the things that we believe might happen, we not only spend time and energy in attracting that result to us, we also hinder ourselves from reaching success. Therefore, if you are worried, honour this emotion by trying to focus on a solution or place your energy into meditation and energy work to resolve the issue. Also, worry is related to fear and fear is the thing that prevents most people from living according to their life purpose.

Gratitude: Being thankful for everything: for each second of life, for the world we live in, for our friends and our families, for our abilities, etc., ensures that we acknowledge how wonderful all these aspects of life are. By doing this, we also make it very clear that we want more of the same and receive additional things that create success and leave us feeling fulfilled.

Work: The work that Usui is referring to is not professional work, but the work we are passionate about. He is reminding us of our life purpose and teaching us that when we live life according to our life purpose we are aligned with Shinki; the Divine. This is how we achieve enlightenment, by creating legacy, investing time in things that we love, and striving to manifest what we are personally passionate about.

Dharma: This is a concept that is so needed in society, but has mostly been forgotten. Dharma is respect for one's teachers—meaning those who inspire us, rather than 'formal' teachers (although this can include formal teachers who inspire you!). When we do not respect the person who teaches us, we cannot respect their teachings either. Nurturing a sense of Dharma for those who guide us through life, helps us gain greater understanding of what they have taught us.

Kindness: Being kind to others, even those who hurt or take advantage of us, keeps us in a healthy place. Hating those who cause us pain, even when that pain is all-consuming, places us in the realms of hatred (not them). Hatred has a very destructive influence on the human being and can cause severe dis-ease. When you feel hatred, you're 'in it' and it is affecting you—turn hatred into kindness and, regardless of the other person, you will be nurturing your own health and wellbeing. Additionally, the people we encounter in our life are merely reflections of ourselves and represent qualities within us. By showing kindness in every part of our life, we are showing kindness to ourselves.

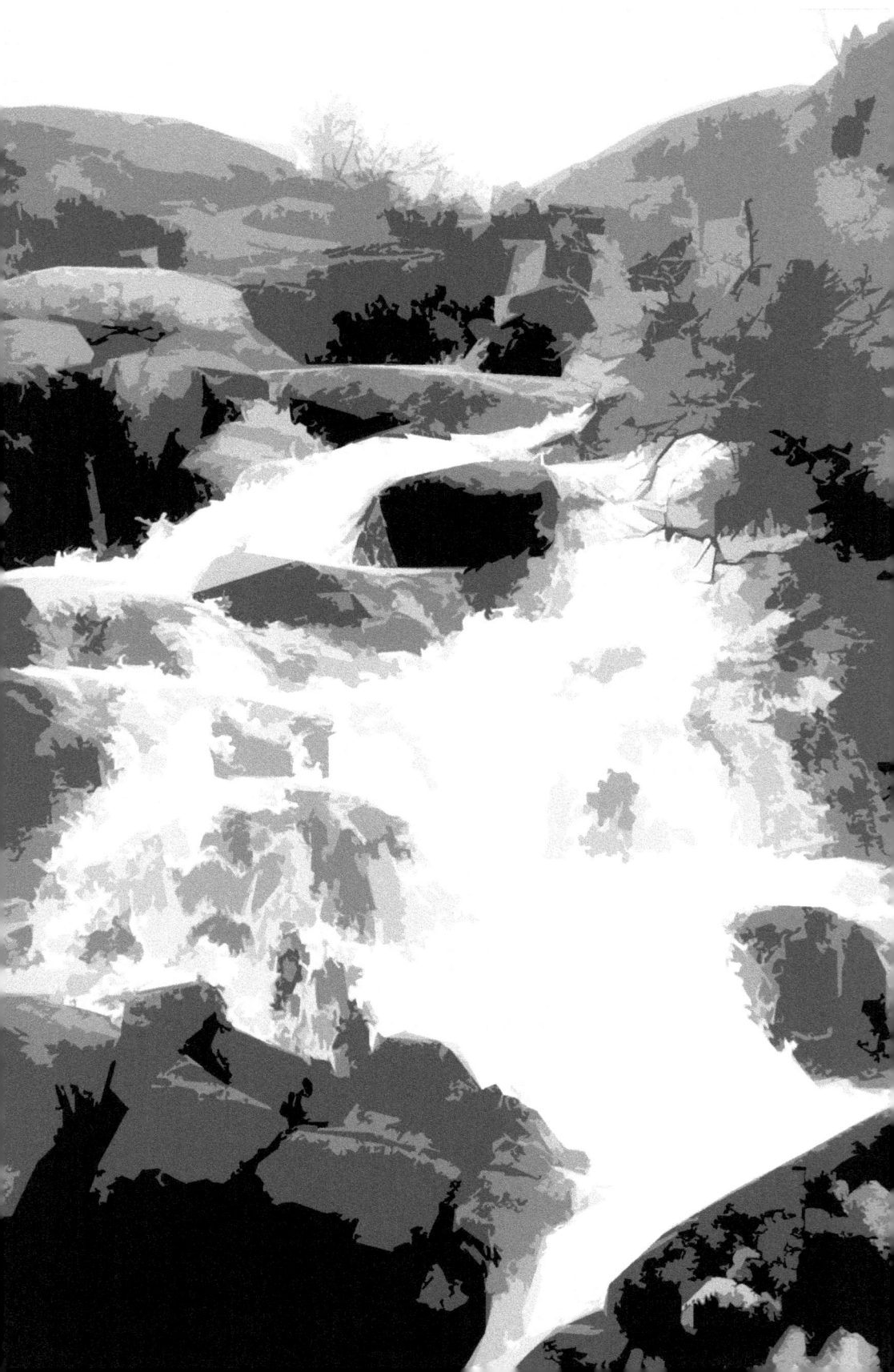

Stepping onto the Path

Whenever you begin on the path of a Reiki modality apprenticeship, one of the first conundrums is how to experience something that so many will never know their entire lives? A mystical force that is simply beyond the awareness of our usual, waking consciousness, can seem so elusive as to be impossible. Yet many Eastern Arts were created and honed over centuries to do just that; to enable those who do not yet know the experience of Ki to grasp it and eventually master their understanding of it.

And, your first experience of a Reiki interaction is very, very special. Just like seeing your favourite movie for the first time, it stays with you; one might say that it 'haunts' you (in a good way!). I believe that our first interaction remains for a long time, and we simply revisit that interaction from our continually evolving perspective—until we have mastered that interaction and are ready for the next.

In vReiki, we have a very specific method for shifting consciousness to the layers of Reiki experiences. This method involves two practices—one conducted by the vReiki Master and the other by their Apprentice (or the Adventurer, as we say in The Reiki Revolution). Both sides of the practice are conducted in tandem and are known as Orientation and Calibration. Before we explore these, however, let us take a moment to discover the historical context of these powerful techniques.

Originally coined as 'empowerments' by Mikao Usui, and nowadays commonly known as 'attunements', Orientations are an alternative way of teaching people how to interact with Reiki and other facets of Ki. Usui based his original empowerments on very ancient practices, reported to have been used by mystics for many thousands of years. Undergoing many evolutions over time, the Orientations of this *Home Experience* are very different in ritual to both the original and Western attunements used in Usui Reiki. They work by 'attracting a person's awareness' to the region of their psyche where a conscious interaction with Reiki can take place. Their interest peaked, it is then the role of the apprentice to focus their experience of the interaction until it becomes a part of their core-being (this is the second stream of the process and known as 'Calibration').

Orientations are still a relatively mysterious process, yet we can appreciate the integral powers at work within the process more than ever before in a modern context. The best metaphor to describe the nature of Orientation is to imagine that you are speaking with somebody who had never seen the colour blue—how would you describe this to them in words so that they could understand what you mean? It is a rather challenging task! However, if you could show them a piece of blue-coloured paper, they would instantly know what blue is and they would never forget it. This is how the Orientation introduces one to the perception of Reiki interactions (interactions that have almost been transpiring, but never before consciously recognised and guided with volition).

Similar to riding a bike, the vReiki Orientations you Calibrate to as part of the *Home Experience* will never be forgotten and can always be recalled even if you haven't practised for many years. It does take a while to integrate fully as a practice, and the wisdom of what these interactions are, will take time to master, however the actual interaction begins instantly and is rather akin to a light switch turning on in your consciousness.

As this happens, you may notice that the effects, or synaesthesia, begin with a subtly profound experience and increase in potency over time, becoming stronger certainly over the three weeks after your have initially Calibrated. Of course, the more you Calibrate to the Orientation, the deeper your understanding will become, and the greater your achievements will be.

As you will be aware, vReiki is taught in six stages. These are Foundation (Zero), Introduction (One), Practitioner (Two), Mentor (Three), Master (Four), and Seer (Five). These degrees of study and mastery were originally introduced so that an apprentice could gradually create a relationship with Reiki at different layers of interaction and perspective. As people have further developed 'transpersonally', the integration has become much smoother and intuitive, meaning that the emphasis on why we need degrees has shifted slightly.

The main reason for these distinctions now is reliant on the purpose you wish to interact with Reiki for. Home use and use on family and friends is covered at this (and the previous) level, professional practice is explored at degree two, and consultancy at degree three. If you want to teach vReiki, then you can explore deeper our adventure, to degree four and once you wish to go beyond the teaching skills of the vReiki Master to work on the advanced spiritual aspects of vReiki, then the Seer Degree (five is now available. At each degree, the Orientations exist at a greater layer of expansion, deeper levels of consciousness, and align further to the Ishiki experience.

Over time you may notice some strange sensory experiences related to your Calibration; these internal experiences can range from subtle distortions in perception, to mesmerising aural/visual displays, intricate and profound messages of wisdom, to very tangible physical sensations. Collectively, these and other similar experience are known as synaesthesia, which relate to an 'overlapping of sensory feedback'. Synaesthesia is when you experience the sensation of one sense, based on the feedback of another.

The most common form of synaesthesia is Visual/Kinaesthetic (VK) Synaesthesia, which can involve effects such as: experiencing pain when watching another person injuring themselves, or experiencing joy upon seeing the colour red. VK Synaesthesia could also be responsible for the awe-inspiring colours, shapes, and visions we experience, as messages from the nervous system are translated by the brain into an extraordinary visual language. Through this language we can interpret our perspective of Reiki and the interactions we are encountering with it.

Other people may hear music, voices, tones, or other sounds that also provide some form of message, pertaining to our interactions with Reiki. There are also people who have kinaesthetic (feeling) synaesthesia; for example, the sensation of falling, spinning, tumbling head over heels, flying, or somebody touching them at different points on their body. Emotional feelings are also very likely to accompany other forms of synaesthesia.

Most people are able to differentiate between their synaesthesia perception and regular perception, however there are people who cannot distinguish the two and experience a synaesthesia effect as 'real'. This can be disconcerting at first, but will soon become vey pleasurable.

When the interaction with Reiki affects your body, resulting in synaesthesia, it is an amazing means of developing your skills as a vReiki Practitioner, Mentor, or Master. And, whilst the reason that you experience these changes is due to your brain trying to understand the complex experience of Reiki, you can use the colours, shapes, sounds, tastes, smells, etc., to piece together some amazing insights into the nature of the Divine. Reiki literally teaches us, through our own phenomenal physiology, how to comprehend divine wisdom.

Common effects of synaesthesia include:

- Brightly coloured flashes of light
- Shapes and movement in front of the eyes
- Distortions, such as that caused by looking through heat
- Strobe effects
- High pitched tones/tinnitus
- Rapid tapping inside the ear, as if a moth is flying about inside
- Inexplicable smells/perfumes that last only for a moment
- Peculiar tastes in your mouth
- Strange feelings of emotion
- Tingling, especially in the head, hands and feet
- Heat in hands, feet or head
- Pins and needles
- Trembling or spasms
- Imagery and 'random' thoughts
- Emotional outbursts

- Headaches or cold/flu-like symptoms
- Extremes of heat and cold
- Magnetic pulling/pushing in hands or body
- Vibrations/trembling sensations, especially in the spine
- The feeling of being touched or prodded
- Flying, falling, spinning, etc.
- People moving around the room
- Psychic-style or intuitive phenomena

These are just some of the sensory experiences you may find after your initial Calibrations to the Orientations of vReiki One; however do not be surprised if you have other effects not mentioned here. These are all natural processes and are in no way detrimental to you. They will enhance your conscious life in so many ways and become a trusted means of experiencing layers beyond our usual senses.

Everybody has a unique way of experiencing synaesthesia and I personally believe that everybody has the ability to consciously recognise synaesthesia—albeit an ability that has rather atrophied in most people. Some people tend to 'see' more, others 'feel', 'hear', or 'taste', and so on. We also tend to have preferences as to which modality we would like to experience. When you do connect to your synaesthesia for the first time, enjoy the moment, even if it is not exactly the type of synaesthesia you wanted! It is very important not to dismiss any synaesthesia, because your brain learns to filter it out very quickly. However, if you focus on your unique experiences, you'll have more of them and they will transform into a multi-sensory experience of synaesthesia, which is even more mind-blowing!

Synaesthesia plays a very important role in the experience of treatments, consultation, and the training methods, however there is much more to our experience of vReiki Mastery than the sensory effects. The role we play in essentially developing an intimate experience of Reiki for ourselves to the level where we feel confident to guide others to their own experiences is at the heart of Mastery. Nowhere is this bond between Master and Apprentice seen as much as in how the Orientations and Calibration philosophy changes our traditional view of discovering Reiki.

The traditional empowerments and 'attunements' of Usui Reiki rely on the Usui Reiki Master 'doing something' to their student; usually manipulating them in some way through the ritual of attunement. The onus is on the Master to create a change in the student. The student closes their eyes, relaxes, and does very little else as part of the experience. For me, this is a very passive approach to interacting with Reiki, which is why I developed the Orientation and Calibration process. When Calibrating, the Apprentice plays an active role in heightening their encounter.

Orientation is like showing The Apprentice a gateway to wonderful new realms of experience. Calibration is the choice the Apprentice makes to go through that gateway, followed by the proactive steps taken to actually do this.

During the process, we use audio companions that play like a movie soundtrack; altering with mood and activity. This is a constant reminder to the Apprentice to maintain their Calibration activities and presents them with a mechanism to propel their synaesthesia to even greater heights of wonder. The narration on these audio companions, or the voice of your vReiki Master in live events, guides you through the various stages of the Orientation and how to best Calibrate.

The ideas of Orientation and Calibration are in real contrast to the more traditional approach to Reiki practice, as are many of the other elements we shall encounter. The best way of understanding how vReiki practices differ from Usui Reiki Ryoho is to explore the standard view of Reiki practices first and then compare these to the vReiki techniques. We interact with Reiki in many different ways for the purpose of achieving satori, or connection to the Divine. The ways of working with Usui Reiki tools include meditation, empowerment, and healing, both with the self and with others.

Traditionally, the procedures in Usui Reiki were based on the practice of Kiko, a graceful series of exercises designed to cultivate reserves of Ki/Chi. The elegant movements made in Kiko act to 'circulate' Ki smoothly throughout your body, releasing any 'blockages' and bringing things into balance on all levels. When discussing traditional views, it is vital that we recognise the difference in the terminology and conceptualisation between the two modalities. In vReiki we transcend the 'linear' concept of 'flow', yet when referring to the historical approach, this is acceptable.

The objective of Usui Reiki practice, as with Kiko, is that, if you can harmonise Ki, you are placing your body in the best possible situation to heal itself on all levels: physical, emotional, mental and spiritual. Kiko practitioners can spend 10–20 years of regular practice to get to Master level, whereas the Usui Reiki ethos is that this can be achieved immediately via the 'attunements'. By forming this connection to Reiki, practitioners can then 'project' Reiki to specific goals, circumstances, to the self for self-healing or others for holistic treatments.

Traditionally, Reiki is understood to travel through the body (via Ki channels known as meridians) and then emanates from the body, especially through the hands, eyes, mouth and feet. 'Reiki projection' is also concentrated around the head and spine. Reiki is often guided to treat physical issues from headaches, backaches, injuries, diseases, chemical imbalances, etc., and can also be used to treat emotional and mental issues as well as life situations and everyday problems including addictions.

Reiki treatments can be created safely and effectively for anybody, ranging from older people to small children and babies. It can help animals, plants and even improve the taste of food and drink. This does mean that an understanding or belief in Usui Reiki techniques is not needed to achieve good results, as one can literally 'taste the difference'!

Those participating in Reiki practice may often experience effects that the interaction with Ki tends to produce in many people, regardless of the reason they have come for treatment. These effects include feelings of calmness and serenity, an ability to cope better with a more positive outlook and be less affected by stress. You may begin to notice these effects yourself once you have Calibrated to the vReiki perspective. There is commonly a definite and noticeable difference in the way you feel about things.

It is traditional within Usui Reiki to think in terms of a 21-day period of clearing or cleansing process as the Ki starts to increase your wellbeing as its first priority. This process is often called an Energy Alignment Process and the effects can appear at any time during the three-week period, although they often last only a few days, to a week. Regular feedback is that of cold and flu-like symptoms, headaches, or feeling quite tired and sleepy. Emotional ups and downs are quite widespread and you may find that you are seeing things in Technicolor for a while, with colours taking on an amazing intensity.

When you first practise interacting with Reiki, it is likely that you will feel simple tingling or heat from your hands with no discernible variation in its intensity. With practice you will develop more sensitivity in your hands and you will be able to feel variations or changes in the sensations you experience. This is because we have a lot of nerves in the hands, so they tend to be a more sensitive area for us to sense the interactions. Although experiences increase in intensity over time, some people are quite sensitive from the first moment: there is a lot of individual variation.

Occasionally you may find that your hands ache when interacting with Reiki; often this is connected with lifting your arms up and holding them in a set position for extended periods —we do get used to it eventually! In some rare circumstances, you may find you feel nauseous when interacting with Reiki. This is often associated with emotional trauma that has become 'dislodged'. The change has caused you to have recognised the trauma and it is a wonderful sign that you are removing the issue at a deep level of being.

So, if this is the usual experience of traditional Usui Reiki and the Western equivalent, how is vReiki any different? Well, now we have had a whirlwind tour of the historical context, the philosophy, and the results this may produce, let us turn our focus to the leading-edge principles of vReiki.

People once thought the Earth was flat and that, if you were to travel far enough, you would eventually fall off the edge.

It was then hypothesised that the Earth was actually a spherical shape that orbited the sun. This new perspective was met with abhorrence and sheer disbelief until it was later proven to be true. This is just one example of how our perception (i.e.: what we see and feel) can deceive us. The world looked flat so therefore it must be flat! The question remains that not many of us have actually witnessed a spherical planet ourselves. We have seen pictures and film footage; some of us have travelled to the other side of the world, but how many have actually travelled so far from the Earth that they can say they have seen the 'round world' with their own eyes? Not many. The fact is that we take this on trust because it is what we are told to believe.

We are told from a very early age to believe only in what we sense with our five 'accepted' senses. Hence we develop into sceptical adults that on one hand believe only what we see and touch, while on the other we trust what we are told, even though we have never experienced it for ourselves. This results in an attitude of mistrust and doubt, whilst living life through the views and perceptions of others.

In the realm of energy medicine, we start from the premise of Ki, which completely defies what we perceive and have been told. Once we begin to understand Ki from our own perspective and release our misgivings, we become unwilling to alter our views again for fear of losing what we have found. Yet the Universe, and the energy from which it is created, never rests or stays the same; it is constantly changing and evolving. We start with the idea that energy can be directed to a point or place because this it what it 'feels' like and that is the way energy works—look at electricity for example!

In recent years the way we perceived Ki started to change and we noticed major repercussions in everyday life. As people became unable to interact with Ki in the way they always had done before, problems began to arise. The issue here was that the majority of people were completely unaware that they had ever been connected to Ki or even that there was such a thing! So we noticed a major shift towards the need to understand more about 'life' and what it is all about. There was a huge increase in people concentrating on complementary medicine, psychic development or a more holistic approach to life.

We also saw an increase in shocking disasters, such as the bombing of the Twin Towers and the London Underground, the Tsunamis of the Indian Ocean and Japan, and so on. These events of mass destruction and death are often ascribed to the changes we are encountering as the Universe evolves. In an attempt to make sense of the terrible things that have happened in the world since the Millennium, we have looked to the wisdom of old soothsayers and prophets who predicted many of the recent events.

A key time in this process began shortly after the millennium with a major shift in our perception of Ki. This shift heralded our introduction to the 'Viridian Age'. As with all transitions, this period may be difficult at times yet is also very rewarding as we learn and evolve into enlightened beings. The Viridian Age is not so much about a change in the energy of the Universe; it is about a change in the way we view that energy/ Ki. It could be seen as the energetic equivalent of moving from a 'flat' view of energy, to a 'spherical' view. In fact the idea of a flat line and a sphere of energy is a very good place to instigate our understanding of Ki from a 'Viridian perspective'.

The traditional view of Ki/Universal Energy perceives life force as flowing from one place to another: this process is often referred to as 'channelling'. Even when we 'channel' Reiki to more than one place (such as in a 'Reiki Triangle') we are still creating a 'flat' line of Reiki. In the Viridian Age we can alter this perspective to where we see ourselves at the centre of a sphere and every other point in the sphere is a place where one can interact with Ki (or other facets of energy/force). This means that in vReiki, we do not channel Reiki from here to there, we directly interact with Reiki at any given point or points. Now on the face of things, this may seem like a simple technicality, however this view gives us a scope and range of techniques that was previously unimaginable.

One simple way of explaining the difference between the Usui Reiki methodology and the vReiki system is that, when you treat a person (or yourself) in the traditional ethos, you create a path from disease to wellbeing. If the treatment subject finds that without their disease they need to take responsibility for an aspect of themselves (such as personal power, fear of the unknown, etc.), they may actually 'walk back' along the path from health to ill health and reintroduce the problem or a similar issue. If we interact with Reiki (from the Viridian perspective) and create a state of wellbeing for them, we offer them no path to walk back down. This means that they can either accept their newfound health, or they choose to walk an entirely different path.

By starting to view the world from the perspective of many dimensions instead of a flat surface, we embark on an even more spectacular journey to places where our vReiki Mastery can become more powerful than has ever been possible in the past—all because we change the way we see the world around us!

So how do we achieve the Reiki equivalent of taking a flat line and making a spherical realm? We simply realise that it was always a sphere—we just only ever saw one part of it! By appreciating this, we realise that whenever we perceive a line, it is just one aspect of a whole. With this in mind, we can now revisit Usui Reiki from a Viridian perspective.

In our 'spherical Reiki' practice (vReiki), we can look at the 'linear Reiki' practice (Usui Reiki) in either a traditional sense or a Viridian sense. This means that you can either use the tools and techniques as they have been used in the past or you can update the tools with your new methodology. Eventually, the line perspective will become ineffectual in the evolving Universal shifts that we encounter but, during this transition, you may find it useful to practise the old and new in tandem. By doing this you will experience the changing Universe for yourself, comprehending at an energetic level how the changes are affecting you and everybody around you.

Mikao Usui developed his self-mastery system based on years of study and satori, the latter connecting him to a higher facet of Ki and the former enabling him to introduce this facet of Ki to others. Hence, they might also achieve satori for themselves. His synthesis of tradition and a new perspective is mirrored in the practice of vReiki, with traditional techniques updated to be more relevant to our ever-evolving Universe.

vReiki is not a 'new and improved' version of Reiki (the force); it is an evolved way of interacting with Reiki. This means the force we experience, i.e.: Reiki, or Ki of the Soul, remains the same, but the way we perceive Reiki and how we express Reiki in the world are evolved to move away from the old linear approach to treatment. Thus we embrace a multidimensional view of the Universe and fuse the old and the new in a way that we can understand and so influence Ki as never before.

This means that many of the old cornerstones of Usui Reiki are preserved, yet in a very different way. Usui commented that the three techniques that comprise the foundation of Usui Reiki Ryoho are Gassho/HatsuReiHo (Connection, Power, Focus, Meditation), Byosen Reikan Ho (Sensitivity), and Reiji Ho (Intuition). So, it is now time for you to to explore the foundation techniques of traditional Usui Reiki and how these can be updated to use them in a 'Viridian Method'.

The Mountain Range beckons! If you have not already done so, Calibrate to the first Orientation and then explore further. On your travels, you will experience these cornerstones of Usui Reiki, as well as some rather fascinating, and sometimes, hidden treasures which you can use in conjunction with the techniques listed in the Appendices.

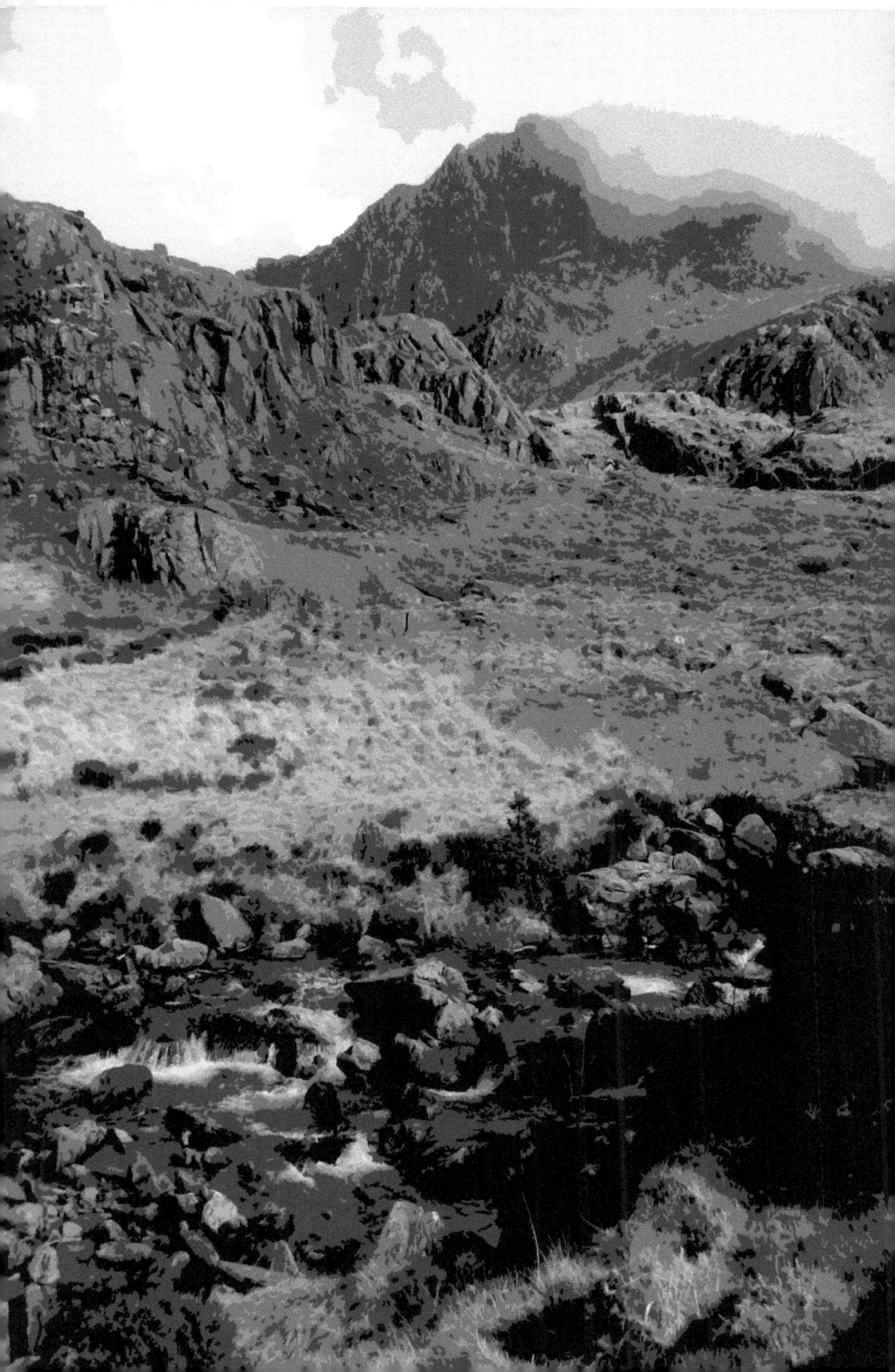

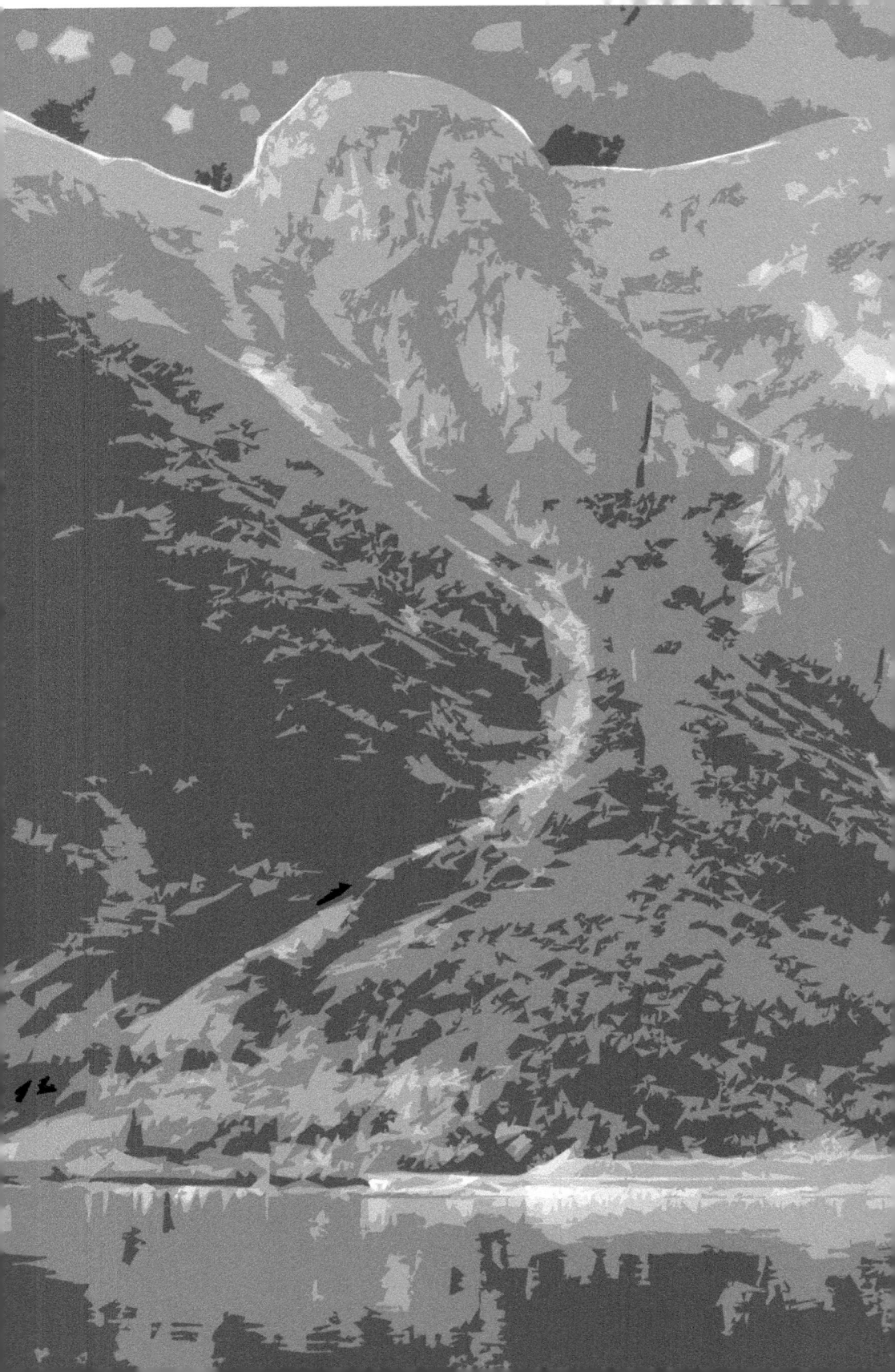

The Moonlit Summit

A Mysterious Light

The lonely traveller walks across the wide moor, her way lit by the cornflower-blue light of the moon. The light is both mysterious and yet, illuminating. For these rays are just enough to light her way, whilst never lifting the cloak of darkness. As this nomad's eyes adjust, over time, to her surrounding, she begins to see more and more of this wild, rugged place; a rock or two, the outline of a gorse bush, a sudden dip in her path. And these are the gifts bestowed upon us by moonlight—it will light our way, but just enough and as we become accustomed to its reflected light, what was once hidden, is revealed.

The force of Tsuki is usually regarded as an aspect of the Intelligent Force; or to explain this in more accurate terms, Tsuki has never been defined outside of vReiki Mastery. Most Masters of Usui Reiki or other modalities, simply experience this facet of Ki as they would Reiki, without differentiation or contrast. However, several years after the origination of vReiki, I was noticing a tangible distinction between three discrete perspectives of Reiki.

Firstly, there was the very familiar experience of the Intelligent Force itself; Reiki. Then, came the layers that were of a more expanded perspective—the experience that occurred a mere fraction away from the oneness of the Divine. Here we can know all that there is to know (except total oneness), as a distinct consciousness. This is Ishiki. And finally, there was the conscious perspective; an experience of actively interacting with Reiki; revealing the secrets that are unmasked as part of that experience. When one observes another, there are two; thus for 'something' to be experiencing Reiki, it cannot be Reiki. Hence, Tsuki was presented with definition and a name.

Since that time, Tsuki has developed into an integral layer of vReiki practice. What many could initially deem to be a 'technicality', has come to life through the definition as a distinct entity in its own right. Not only showing us the power of definition, but also revealing the complexity of Ki, in all its enigmatic and hidden depths. Yet it is important to remember that (as with all the facets of Ki) Tsuki is not separate or somehow 'removed'; I did not 'chunk down' to gain an understanding of Tsuki, but instead, sculpted my experience of this Mysterious Light, through the understanding of the intricate relationship between the observer and the observed.

Just as Shinki cannot know itself without some form of separation, albeit illusionary, nobody and nothing can experience itself from a completely external position without becoming 'something else' (which is equally as illusionary). Therefore, we develop the observer and the observed; two distinct facets of oneness that create definition. However, this is merely the beginning of the adventure, because the act of observation, changed the experience of the observed and the observer.

We could imagine this as, Reiki, observing itself as Ishiki and creating a change that we now understand as Tsuki. Or, could it be the physical manifestation of the Divine, Ishiki, observing itself consciously (Tsuki), to create changes that are experienced as Reiki? The Trinity of facets that form Ishiki, Reiki, and Tsuki are all one and yet discrete facets that interact to change the experience of each. Furthermore, when a vReiki Master interacts with one of these three facets, the experience creates new ripples of change that add to the wondrous complexities of our Mastery.

Just as wanderer upon the moor is guided by the moonlight, we are ushered on our journey by Tsuki; the Ki of the Moon. Rather like its namesake, however, Tsuki only reveals a greater degree of experience when we are accustomed to its light. I believe this is why people mostly experience Tsuki as Reiki... they never actually see beyond the initial glance to a deeper understanding of this elusive force. This is expressed on several occasion in *The Reiki Revolution Home Experience*, where Adventurers are invited to search a particular area many, many times before truly understanding subtle differences in what they are investigating.

Tsuki is like an orchestral symphony that requires several listenings before the delicate interplay of the sounds is apparent. Tsuki is an awe-inspiring sunset that creates colours we need to study carefully to recognise. Tsuki is an emotion that is misinterpreted as another, similar emotion, yet offers its own unique drives and passions. Tsuki is the part you play in any vReiki practice, or the part you experience when you are 'at one' with Reiki. So, in a typical treatment, you will transition between the experience of Reiki and Tsuki (and Ishiki) many times—the art of vTsuki Mastery is being able to recognise and express which perspective you have shifted to at any given moment.

Ishiki is the Ki of Consciousness, although this refers to a transpersonal consciousness—in other words it is a Universal consciousness, rather than the conscious experiences of one ego-self. Tsuki, is the conscious experience of one person, which transcends the usual concept we have of a person. For in the Realms of Tsuki, we experience ourselves as many contrasting, and sometimes conflicting, layers of consciousness and perspective. What I class as me, and you as you, are revealed to be a plethora of egocentric viewpoints, all competing for realisation, through conscious focus. The aspects of yourself that you believe to be you, are merely those who have become consciously recognised over time and because of repetition. The dis-eased person, who has yet to realise their healthy layers of being; the person who has 'failed' repeatedly, because of the need to recognise themselves as a huge success; the shy one in the corner, who fears discovering their gregarious and confident self.

Tsuki is our Ki to interaction with all these aspects of ourselves; from the most obvious layers of our psyche, to the repressed and the hidden fragments. Yet, Tsuki will only ever show us enough to guide our way on the journey of the ego-self; it is only with familiarity we will distinguish other aspects of ourselves that we can then heal, enhance, or transform.

When venturing along our path with Tsuki, we encounter many themes that have developed over years of life; themes that have developed beliefs and behaviours. These are the shades of our personality that drive us or hold us back. So, the first area of interaction with Tsuki is that of self-discovery, where we encourage the expansive parts of the self and alter the contractive facets. (The Ishiki blueprint of this adventure is centred around a person uncovering their Core-Self, their passion, and life purpose. For when we know who we are and what we were destined to achieve, we create a wondrous legacy for those to come and fulfil our Shinki vision.)

As we go forward with our Tsuki interactions, we develop a deep sense of knowing and intuitive abilities, rather like the psychic awareness of Jiki, but at a more expanded (less physical) level. To appreciate this fully, interacting with Jiki creates psychic abilities based upon the physical world, events, people, places, etc. Tsuki intuition is more 'Universal', with a sensitivity to evolutionary shifts in the perception of humankind, the ever-changing awareness of Earth-self, and knowledge of hidden wisdom.

Connected very deeply to the subconscious, Tsuki interactions can produce a deep resonance with subtle-layers of experience—the Earth, different 'dimensions' or aspects of consciousness, the stars, the Universe. This presents us with the ability to create a profound healing of the Earth-self, very tangible communication with Mystics and other sentient beings, as well as a greater sense of the vastness/minuteness of all things. If Ishiki is the Divine plan and Reiki, a bridge to the Divine, then Tsuki is our intimate and personal experience of the Divine... and as the Divine.

Just as Tsuki is sculpted from Reiki, it also contains aspects that are a continuation, or expression of Jiki. As all facets of Ki exist as one, whilst maintaining a discreet identity of their own, the blending of the regions between Reiki and Jiki, is the experience of Tsuki. Like a human face, the nose becomes the cheek, the cheek flows into the chin; each feature has its own identity and traits, yet each is an integral part of one face. As the features of a face can be experienced in a focused stare, isolated by the transitions surrounding them, we can equally enjoy the beauty of an entire face, by softening the transitions to create a vision of wholeness. This applies to Ki also; for Tsuki could be the jawline or the brow, it may be the way light and shadow interact, a flush of colour or delicate texture, it can express a million emotions, or display the wrinkles and lines of an age-gleaned wisdom.

This blending between definition and oneness (the sculpting of Ki through human experience), is a foundation to the way different facets of Ki interrelate so magnificently in treatment, consultation, ritual, and strategy. It is why a single technique can be interchanged to interact with different facets of Ki; how many facets can be interacted with, through just one methodology. And why, at any given moment, there are usually various facets interacting with us—we merely focus on the predominant facet that is attracting our awareness at that time.

With this in mind, it is Tsuki interactions (often in tandem with Jiki) that present us with a flare for consultation, planning, and more 'cerebral' aspects of vReiki Mastery. As we shall investigate later in this *Home Experience*, producing a strategy for each client, situation, or particular goal we have, helps us sculpt an effective plan without straying from our ethos of holism. Too often in treatments and practices, old habits can lead to highlighting symptoms (and thus treating at a surface layer of being). An effective and multi-dimensional sculpture of how to proceed will keep reminding us of the Core-Self Shinki that we strive to attain.

The creation of client, business, global, or person plans can be extremely good fun, especially if you like lists and colour-coding! For others, it is the intuitive and 'inner-knowing' aspects of vTsuki that thrill vReiki Masters. For, as we interact with Tsuki on behalf of our clients, etc., consultations can come alive with wonder and the most staggering dialogue. As Master and Apprentice, or Master and client enter into the crucible of Tsuki interactions, their oneness becomes a visceral, corporeal experience, as we present insight into seemingly impossible challenges or solutions to all-encompassing limitations, and they use these to build a way forward into the darkness, guided by that cornflower-blue light.

The Cohesion of Consciousness

To comprehend how Tsuki interacts with us, we need to examine how consciousness 'works' and some of the deeper wisdom that exists around the concept of conscious experience. Whilst science scrambles for answers as to the nature of the conscious mind, our experiences in vReiki can present to us a much more profound and personal solution to the enigma of conscious thought.

Life is made of moments. Seemingly random moments that connect into a lifetime and a legacy. In every moment, we make choices that affect the outcome of one moment and which moment we experience next. You see, each moment is not predetermined or fixed; it is just one in an infinite array of moments; experiences that we can 'step into' and grasp with every fibre of our being. The linear perspective of life as a straight line is merely one aspect of the Shinki's master illusion of physicality. From every moment that is, was, or can be, exists as layer-upon-layer of experience, which is just waiting to happen.

The act of being in a moment is recorded by our brain and converted to memory as we move to the next moment. This means that at any given moment we are having multiple experiences... Being engaged with the moment, experiencing the previous moments we have encountered in short-term memory, those in long-term memory, or pre-empting 'future' moments. In every moment we are presented with a choice; whether to be fully engaged in the here and now, or to access memories/desires, which take us out of the current moment.

To illustrate this, imagine being in a moment that is a 'pinnacle experience'—one of great achievement, joy, or wonder. Here you are fully engaged in the moment and making memories of that moment. Your senses are fully responsive to the stimuli around you and you drink in every aspect of this wonderful experience. In future moments, any one aspect that reminds you of this moment, will trigger the same emotions and behaviour as this one now, thus bringing you out of that moment and into the next.

Conversely, a traumatic memory can cause you fear, anger, or frustration in the moment (even if that moment has little in common with your previous experiences). Here a person might choose not to continue with that moment and to move away from the very thing they are searching for (because they do not like the sensations this set of circumstances is giving them). As an aside, I have seen many students who get so close to their answers and healing, only to jump to a different form of therapy at the crucial moment…. Because they are getting so close to their pain (so that they can transform it), nonetheless, they run away in terror!

For the majority of people, the choices of which moment comes next and the level of engagement in any given moment, happens by default, rather than by design. It is such an unfortunate aspect of being human that, despite how amazing we are, we rarely engage with our fullest potential. Instead we just 'sail along', believing that 'this is it'.

In every moment, success is but a moment away, literally. We can engage in such a way as to plunge into the most awe-inspiring experiences imaginable; except memories often tell us a different story. Hence, we tend towards a life, lived in reminiscence or future dreams, without giving thought to the infinite possibilities at our feet.

This moment, right now, exists in duality—it is the moment in your consciousness and it is also the moment that is actually happening. The two are not the same and never will be. As you move forward, an infinite range of possibilities sits ahead of you; these moments exist in potential and concurrently, each as real as the next. As you choose (with volition or by habit) which step to make, all the moments converge into a single moment. It is this moment that becomes the physical reality and thus, the one you base your conscious experiences upon. This Viridian philosophy has produced miracles right in front me; I have experienced people change their lives in an instant with a true understanding of this principle alone!

It is the passage from moment to moment that creates the line we experience, not the path we walk on. The fact is, there is no path, until we step forward—then the path appears as a symptom of human conditioning. As a vReiki or VM Master, people experience their realities very differently; flipping between the usual concept of physical reality and multi-dimensional experiences that exist beyond that illusion. Both of these states are necessary to function in the physical world, whilst also enriching your life, and those around you, in the most wondrous ways possible.

In addition to this remarkable ethos, there are other layers of experience that also exist in the moment; constantly sitting between us and the world, and also behind the conscious experience of life. These are the facets of ourselves we collectively refer to as the 'subconscious mind'. Here, varying degrees of awareness from 'relaxed' to 'comatose', monitor, distort, erase, and completely change our experiences. These regions of our psyche traverse the bridge between the ego-driven individual and the transpersonal consciousness, and so, incessantly strive to balance our individual desires, fears, foibles, and perspectives, with those of the collective awareness (which leads onto the life purpose blueprint of Ishiki).

Tsuki is the facet of Ki that unlocks the secrets of these subconscious facets of being, as well as guiding us through the momentary aspects of conscious experience. For, whilst we know each moment to be transitory and fleeting, Tsuki knows the eternal nature of moments. Consciously experienced by Shinki, through the illusion of our senses, what we do in the here and now has always existed in potential, transformed into physical reality by our choices, and presented to Shinki, through our own perspective.

For we burst into this life with a purpose to fulfil and a legacy to create. We jump headlong into living and usually come screeching to a halt as we are indoctrinated into our social and cultural prisons. Within each of each is the whole Universe waiting to get out! We are a spark of the Divine; a joyous roller coaster ride of experiences, waiting to happen. Then we settle for some other person's vision of what is 'right' for us. When you discover your Core-Self motivations and live to their inspirational purpose, you learn how to break free of the constraints upon you and to live a remarkable life. This is how Tsuki guides and nurtures you.

In each moment, Tsuki is sculpting your experiences at subliminal layers of consciousness to bring you back to your life purpose. The same circumstances keep happening in different situations; traumas keep arising in contrasting ways, cycles repeat, weird thing happen, strange connections grab your attention, and so on—all Tsuki, beavering away in the background to give you a sense of mission and purpose; to reignite the spark of your passion, whatever that may be.

As an expression of Reiki, yet an autonomous force in its own right, Tsuki sheds enough light upon us in any given moment to light the way forward and to present us with clues, but never to show us the entire picture. To do so would negate personal choice—the most sacred of human characteristics. All intelligent life is blessed with the power of choice, it is what enables us to live with fulfilment and joy, to fall in love, to taste every morsel, and drink thirstily from the ever-abundant cup of experience. Without choice, Shinki could never realise the one thing that created the physical Universe–what it is to not be Shinki!

We are sparks, capricious, fleeting bursts of light that set fires or fade into darkness. Tsuki reminds us to burn brightly, defiant against the shadows we create and focused upon that never-ending flame that is our legacy in making. Interacting with Tsuki, offers us light reflected. Light that is not so bright it blinds and burns, but instead it guides us ever-onwards, ever-knowing that the next step is what we make it...

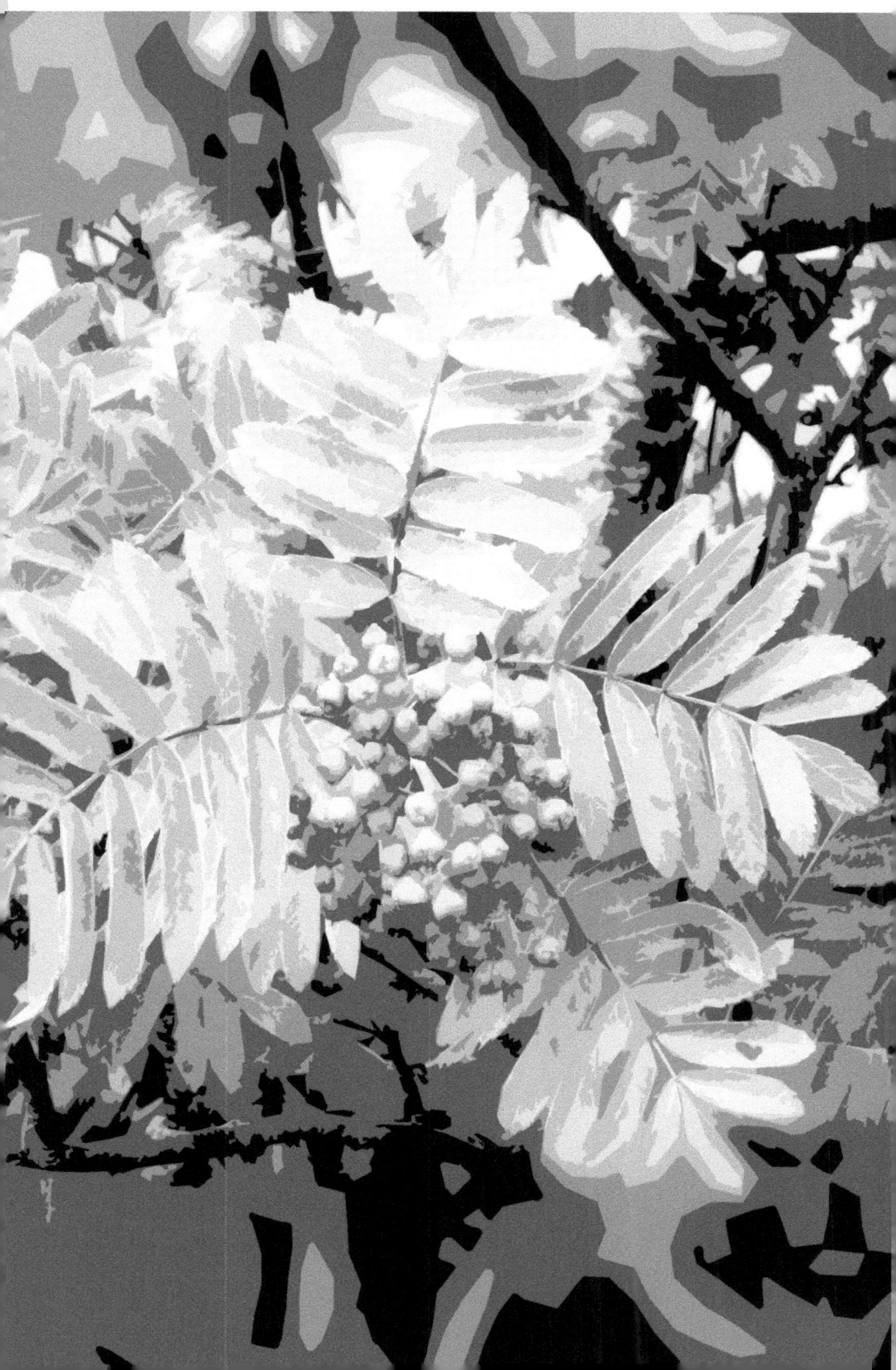

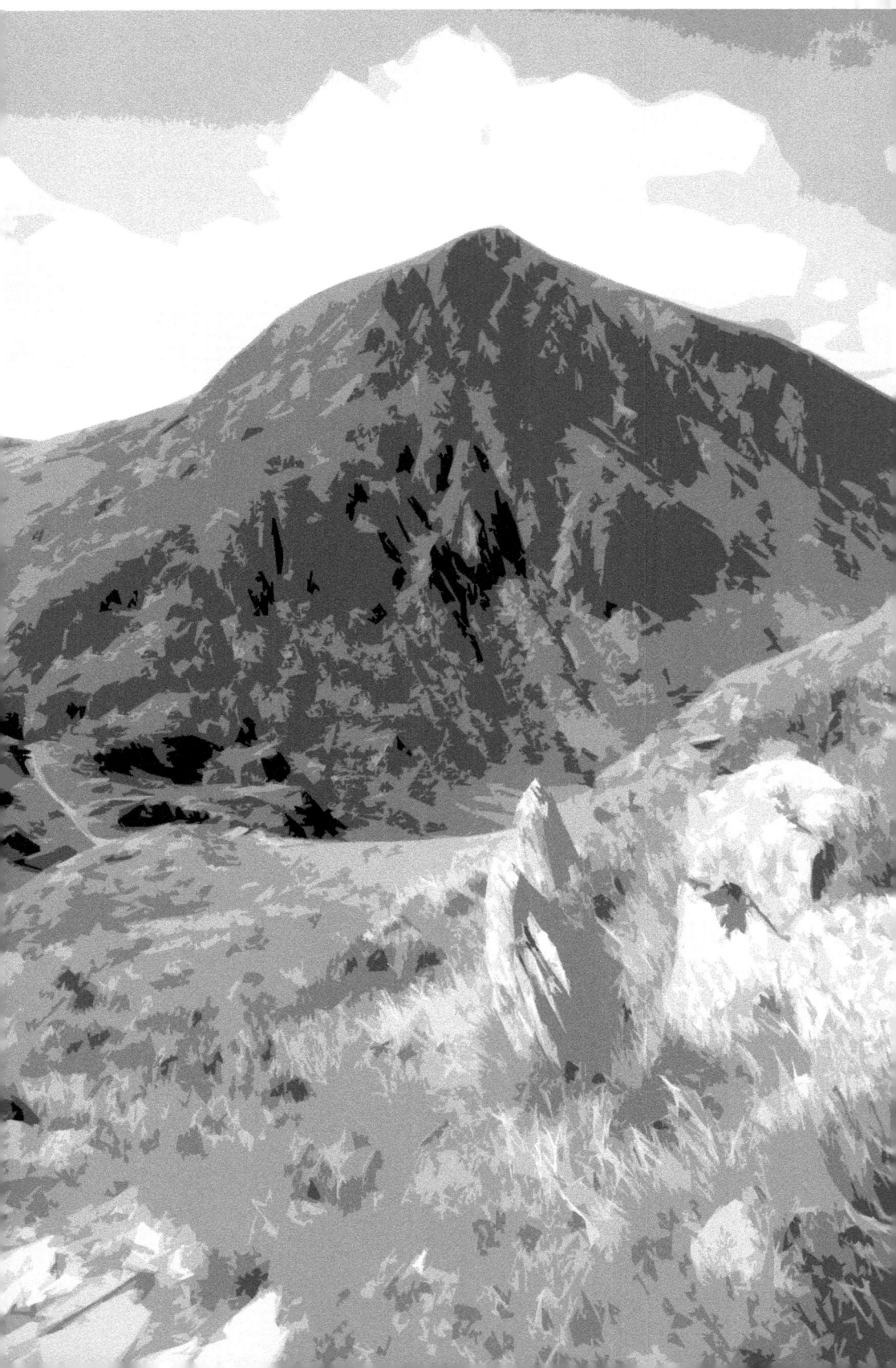

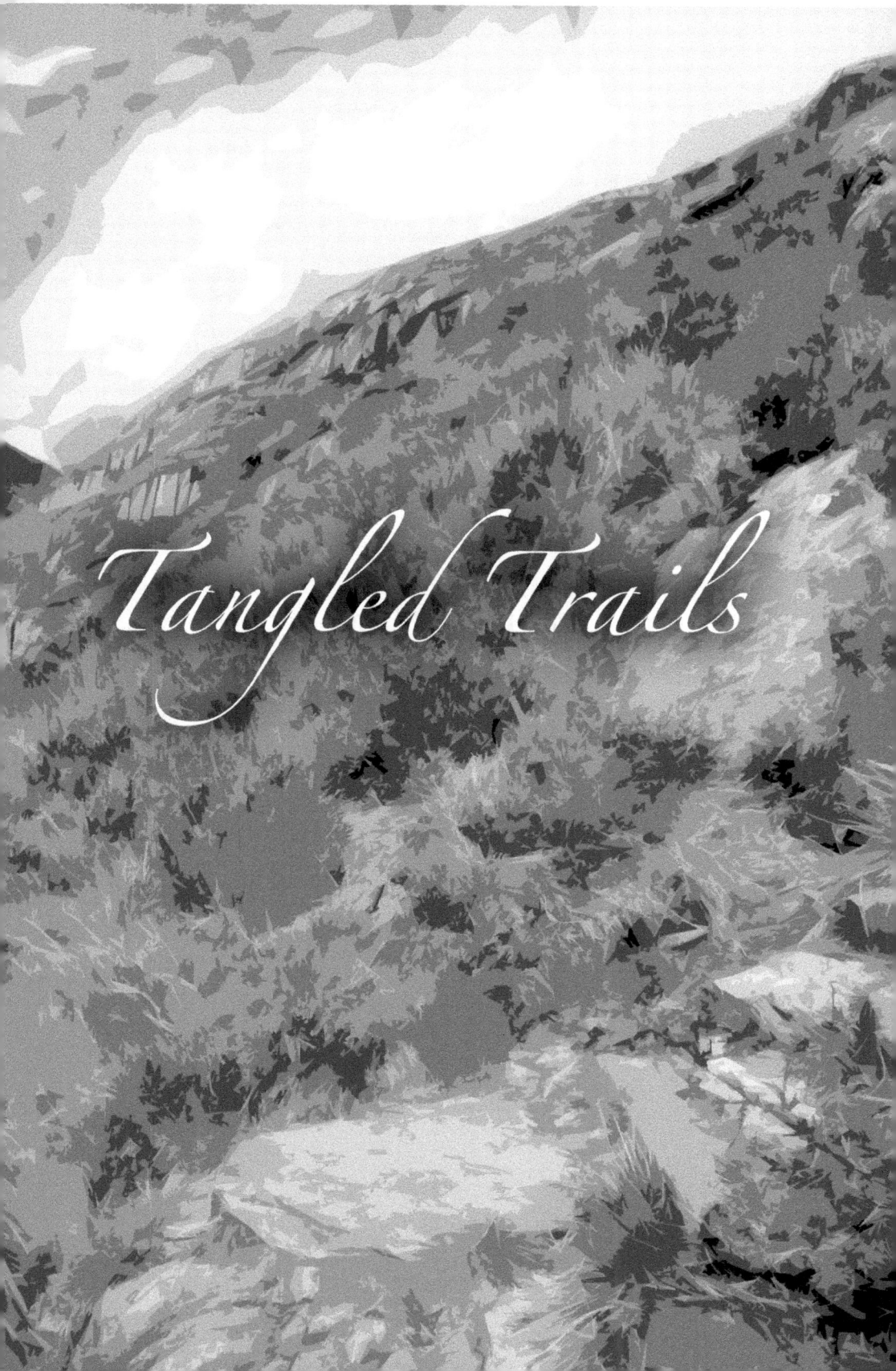

Tangled Trails

A Magnetic Power

Very little is known about Jiki. References to this particular facet of Ki are limited to the teachings of specific philosophers and certain historical documents. The resurrection of Jiki practice was originated unintentionally, while I was attempting to devise a way of teaching people how to activate their psychic senses, using the same method of Orientation as I originated in vReiki practice.

When working with the specific perspective of energy that psychic mediums shift to, I noticed that the experience of this perspective was very magnetic in sensation, which caused me to ponder the mysterious force of Jiki. I knew that Jiki could be interacted with in much the same way as Reiki, however, as no living person has consciously influenced Jiki and written about their experiences under the term, 'Jiki', it was highly improbable that I could ever achieve this feat!

However, my years of experience, originating with energy therapies (such as the Viridian Method) had taught me how to compare the experiences of Ki and of other perspectives of energy. For instance, when interacting with Reiki, I could equate the experiences I had to specific perspectives of energy known as 'Essences'. An Essence is 'the entire Universe, viewed from a single viewpoint' and these are used in Celtic Reiki, VM, and other therapies. I began testing Essences that created similar experiences to Reiki and then adjusted these to match the experiences of Psychic Mediumship. The breakthrough then came, when I applied my own shift in perspective (from the Reiki-like-Essences to the Psychic-like-Essences) to my interactions with Reiki itself. Since then I have been able to interact with Jiki and apply the results extensively through vReiki.

As a facet of Ki that has rarely been explored consciously, the perception of Jiki has been very much new territory for those of us who have experienced it. Yet despite this modern perspective of an age-old life force, I wanted to maintain a degree of tradition in the practice of vJiki while still reflecting the Viridian perspective of our new age.

Therefore, the tools we investigate in this workshop are a mixture of the old; as used in Shinto, Taoist and Buddhist Ki practices, and the new; with Viridian Method philosophies supporting the way we use the aforementioned tools. This means that as well as interacting with Jiki for psychic and manifestation purposes, we can also integrate our experiences with Reiki to enhance our healing skills and systems.

The Japanese word 'Jiki' can be directly translated to the Western concept of magnetic force and the concept of 'magnetic Ki' is derived from the Shinto view of life force. In many respects comparable to the scientific view of an electromagnetic spectrum, the philosophy describes all Ki as divided into facets, some of which are adaptable. Yet when stable they have a specific and definite purpose. As we have seen, these facets range from Shinki to Kekki; Shinki being able to change itself to any other facet of Ki while always remaining Shinki, while the other aspects of Ki interact with each other in complex dynamics.

Whereas Reiki is viewed as the great harmoniser of Ki; the facet that balances with highly superior intelligence and minimum physicality, Jiki is the aspect of Ki that guides us at a group level as well as individually. As people, we are all very different and while we may have much in common with others, we are still unique and individual. With all this contrast and diversity, it would be very easy for us to walk in very different, opposing directions. As each person walks his or her path, they play a part in a huge expansion. An example could be seen as everybody starting in New York and gradually walking forwards in different directions—as this happens the group expands in all directions. When somebody reaches Toronto, somebody on the opposite side of the group arrives at Orlando, and so on.

With all the multiplicity of things in life, from science, to art, to spirituality, to health, to love, to business, to personal tastes, we can connect to an almost endless number of personal choices. Each choice is like a village or town on the map we are travelling. With this much to choose from, it would not be long before we disperse so far from each other that we would just dissipate. It is here where Jiki comes into being, for Jiki creates magnetism in groups; a magnetism that binds us together so that we remain close enough to preserve stability as a race.

All groups interact with Jiki when they begin to disperse as this particular facet of Ki will bring them closer together, while maintaining individuality within the group. This means that we are not only connected to each other through Jiki, but we are also connected to all living things, all places, all events, all planets, all stars, all galaxies, and so on. When Reiki creates harmony and beauty, it is interacting with Jiki to achieve it in the physical world. For, the charismatic Jiki ensures that we work together for the good of all.

As with all magnetism, there is a flip side to the nature of Jiki for, in addition to its attractive properties, it also repels. This means that in group dynamics the same force that keep us together can also push us apart. As Jiki pulls us closer and separates us, we move forward, driven by relationships, interactions, situations and circumstances. In some instances we may be propelled in one direction at an amazing pace, whilst at other times we may meander slowly on a multitude of paths. There are also occasions when we become 'stuck' between two equal and opposing forces. Here we become still, yet because of the huge power of this divergent force, we are buffeted and impacted from both directions.

As a group of individuals each follow their unique needs and create their personal life path, the group begins to expand and separate. The more people run towards their goals, the greater the overall expansion, and so, the divergence continues until the group finally dissipates and no longer exists. Jiki attracts and repels the members of a group, so that the group remains cohesive. Each member of the group can then go their own way, within the loose confines of the whole. Hence the group remains intact and each individual can follow their path at a harmonious pace.

This means that as we interact and move in relation to the overall dynamics of our family, social, community, geographic and biological groups, we will also be influenced by our location within these groups. Those at the centre of the Jiki sphere of authority will move in line with the group, whilst those at the fringes will move in their chosen direction, either leading the group, or opposing the group. Those leading will often be held back while the group 'catches up' and at anytime the group may decide to move in a different direction.

Of course, there are times when an individual disagrees with the group or discovers an 'unconventional' way of doing things. When this occurs, two possible outcomes are available: the individual separates from the group and moves to another 'sphere of reality', or the group likes this 'new' way of doing things and moves with the individual in this new direction. This entire process is done without communication at a conscious level and happens under the natural dynamics of Jiki.

If we examine these dynamics more closely we see that Jiki is, at any given moment, directing a very complex dance of attraction and repulsion. It is moving particular experiences towards us and pushing others away. For the most part these interactions are 'internal workings' and can be seen as superfluous to the overall dynamic. However, when we interact consciously with Jiki, we can not only influence it to a certain extent, but we can also read its dynamics.

The effect we have of consciously entraining the attractions and repulsions is often known as 'manifestation' as we can draw what we want in life towards us and remove the situations/circumstance that we do not want. The reading of Jiki dynamics is known commonly as 'psychic ability'—we not only say what has happened and what is occurring at this moment, but also what is about to take place in the future.

Jiki usually remains on the very borders of consciousness. We are aware of its actions and consequences, but direct (albeit unconscious) interaction with Jiki is usually reserved for those who are said to have special gifts or natural abilities. The perspective of Jiki is actually nearer to our own than that of Reiki so (as people who have Calibrated to the perspective of Reiki often say) Reiki helps us to improve psychic abilities and we can manifest better lives with Reiki Mastery. In actuality, we could say that Reiki is interacting with Jiki to achieve these results and the more people connect to Reiki, the closer they shift their own perspective to the realms of Jiki.

Now to understand how we can actually 'read' and influence dynamics, through our interactions with Jiki (as part of our vJiki practice), we need to examine the interrelation of Ki that exists beyond our physical perception. When we act with any form of Reiki therapy practice, we use our senses to interpret what we are doing and the effect it is having. The problem is that the 'rules' of our physical world are not the same as those of the non-physical or 'potential realms'. So the sensations and actions of energy may appear to be one thing, when actually they are something different.

When we connect to dynamics of a particular type, we entrain to them which means that we start to resonate at the same experiential rate. Now, whilst the Usui Reiki convention is to think about Ki as 'around us', the vReiki methodology asserts that physical location bears no relation to Ki! If you are standing in a room with somebody and you are happy, whilst they are angry, you are in two different states of being. Your experiences need never meet. The challenge is, because they are in our physical space we try to adapt to them and physical entrainment takes place.

As children we can browse through vast realms of experience, connecting to many different realities and realms, yet we are soon trained into physical 'reality', where we automatically entrain to our surroundings (which to some extent is necessary for the survival of the physical body, although years of dogma have distorted our education into moral or psychological entrapment). This is why we forget our natural abilities and massive wealth of energetic power. If ever you observe children playing, listening to a story, or watching a cartoon, you will see that they can be completely absorbed by the energy of it; as if they are somewhere else completely. This is the skill that we lose as adults.

However, we do not need to interact with the experience and dynamics of our physical space, for at anytime, we are free to shift to another realm; a totally different perception or interaction with Ki. When we do entrain to the experience of our choosing, we become that experience. In other words, as we saw earlier, Ki does not simply pass through us as water through a drainpipe; we become intrinsically woven into the facet of Ki and its immense power.

The Dynamics of Intuition

Whenever we interact with Jiki, we activate an awareness of the dynamics from which the physical world is created and, in the same way as we can focus upon an aspect of ourselves, we can hone in on the elements of these 'Jiki dynamics' as we choose to. We entrain to and so become Jiki, by experiencing Jiki on a greater scale. We do this by monitoring the synaesthesia we consciously experience, whilst interacting. Jiki is an expression of us, so we can change our perspective or thoughts to create changes within the Jiki and then read those changes back.

In everyday terms this can be translated to extra-sensory perception, or intuitive ability. By using Jiki, we can perceive the changes and realignment of energetic patterns and we do this 'outside' the physical parameters of space and time which are, after all, artificial concepts and do not actually exist outside of our human perception. By examining a specific dynamic (an attraction or repulsion) of Jiki, we can gain an insight into what is happening at a subtle level of Universal interaction and how this translates into physical reality.

Another way of understanding this concept is to imagine all the different dynamics that Jiki is an integral part of at any given time. At each and every moment, Jiki is an expression of groups from the very small, to the inconceivably massive and how each of us interact as part of those communities. By connecting to Jiki and entraining to the same experiential rate, you bring into your awareness all of these dynamics and will automatically concentrate on the ones that have the most relevance to you at that moment. In this way you can perceive the dynamics that are occurring within Jiki and interpret these into our way of physically viewing the world.

The particular technique for enhancing our intuitive abilities depends very much on your connection to it—the stronger you can integrate with Jiki, the better you will be able to interpret and influence it. And, to assist you on this path, various tools and techniques are available in the virtual Realms of the *Home Experience*.

When using your intuitive or psychic abilities, your main 'tool' is your body, emotions and mind—and the synaesthesia they produce. However you choose to interact in any given environment or practice will dictate how much information you receive as well as the clarity and accuracy of that information. Therefore, the key to psychic training using Jiki is regular practice that you can use in your everyday life which will help you develop your body and mind's natural abilities to sense what is usually hidden and beyond the realms of perception. The areas of focus when working with Jiki and the aspects of you that respond to psychic development training are:

- Clearing and Healing
- Raised Awareness and Focus
- Increased Sensitivity
- Intuitive Ability
- Imagination and Descriptive Skills
- Assertion and Confidence

Once you have started to develop your vJiki practice, you will find that a whole range of new and exciting activities are available to you. These can include some of the practices covered in this *Home Experience*, but remember that potential for Jiki interactions is unlimited, and you can take the main focus of your psychic abilities wherever you want. Some suggestions for regions that might interest you are:

- Mystic Work
- Communication with Spirits, Ghosts, and other Entities
- Lost Soul Work
- Intuition and 'ESP'
- Psychometry
- Personal Readings
- Karmic Regression and Past-Life Readings
- Vibrational Healing

Developing your sensory skills in order to understand the subtle information embedded within the dynamics of Jiki and perceiving other levels of being can be an exciting and rewarding exercise, yet as with Reiki-based healing practices, psychic development also requires regular effort and a commitment to evolve as a person from a core passion. Whilst some people do retain varying degrees of psychic ability from childhood, most of us have to relearn how to use our synaesthesia-sensory abilities.

Psychic ability is not really about 'seeing ghosts', although this is very often the aspect of it that catches the imagination. Psychic ability is about developing your senses to perceive the world around you in a different way; whether that is working with the subtle information, expressed through the location or objects in it, helping people with therapeutic Reiki treatments, personal readings and past-life information or sensing beings that do not have much physical form. If working with Reiki practice encompasses healing, self-mastery and enlightenment, Jiki practices are sensory, communicative and intuitive.

Very often, the first step in evolving your psychic senses is to leave behind any preconceived ideas about what you think is going to happen and practising techniques that sometimes appear to bear no relation to the end result! In fact, psychic training can be compared to how Operatic Performers develop the ability to sing, which often means they do not sing for long periods in favour of breathing exercises and abdominal fitness training!

There are several steps in a psychic development regime, which we now explore as different aspects of the process. These could be viewed as linear progression to your development, though in the majority of instances, these stages will be concurrent and interrelated.

Clearing and Healing

This initial stage of the psychic training process is integral to evolving yourself to the required level of sensory health. When using the subtle information that mediums use, we need to interact with Jiki in a particular way: this often means that we need to raise the perception of our senses and deepen our synaesthesia experiences.

If you have had trauma or emotional upheaval in your past, this can hinder the ability to expand your awareness to the necessary layers of consciousness. Therefore, many cannot connect to Jiki and experience the wonder of its dynamics. The underlying experiences of fear, anger, grief, hatred, jealousy and so on, all stop us shifting to the perspective associated with psychic ability.

These experiences (of fear, anger, and so forth) are associated with unpleasant memories or pain and tend to distract us from the task at hand. When experiencing these emotions and reliving the memories attached to them, it can be very challenging to see beyond them and to the 'place' where we interact with Jiki. So the more you can remove your associations to these emotions and therefore, lessen the frequency of their presence, the more you will perceive in your sensory synaesthesia.

vReiki treatment methods are an excellent way of assisting this process, which is often why Reiki practitioners report enhanced psychic and intuitive abilities. Our perception of Reiki, requires a greater degree of conscious expansion than it takes to recognise Jiki, so by interacting with Reiki on a regular basis, we become adept at a level of expansion that makes interaction with Jiki very easy.

Raised Awareness and Focus

Raising your awareness of the dynamics you encounter could be viewed as an extension to the healing and clearing processes previously discussed, as it continues the expansion of your conscious awareness. When you cast aside the habitual contraction that occurs when you experience painful memories and unrelinquished trauma, you expand your perception to a level where you interact with wiser, less physical facets of Ki (which, in turn, lift you further).

To understand the processes of psychic development better, we could use the analogy of a person trying to climb a cliff-face where the bottom is the starting point and the top is a state of proficiency in psychic ability. They start up the cliff with a rucksack on their back which is filled with heavy pieces of rock. These could be seen as their painful emotions and trauma. As they drop each rock, they weigh less and climbing the cliff is easier. Having dropped many rocks, they start to expand their awareness, which could be viewed as using helium-filled balloons to make them lighter. These balloons can actually lift our climber up so high that they no longer need to climb—they simply float upwards to their goal!

Another aspect of vJiki training that goes hand-in-hand with the raising of awareness is that of focus. Without the ability to focus completely on our experiences of Jiki interactions, we are often too distracted by other factors to glean any valuable information. Some people find the inability to focus on what they are doing so strong that it actually hinders their development and they give up trying. Here, a person's awareness is habitual trained 'out there', and not upon the internal synaesthesia and feedback of intuition. When learning to focus intently and for long periods, remember to turn inwards – to your core—and remain 'thought-free' until you experience the feedback you want.

Increased Sensitivity

Once you have started to interact with Jiki using your own volition, the next step is recognising that you have done so. This is another area where people often need help in their training, as preconceived ideas of what they 'should' be 'seeing' or 'feeling', detract from their inner-synaesthesia experiences. Dismissing synaesthesia as 'imagination' or second-guessing it when recognised is guaranteed to make it disappear surprisingly quickly. This is because we are so accustomed to 'filtering out' synaesthesia from our awareness that to do so, comes very naturally to us. Yet, to grow your intuitive abilities, you need to have faith that it is a very real phenomena.

Gradually, this will build your evolving sensitivity to the point where synaesthesia is all-embracing for you.

The initial stages of your psychic enhancement may present you with vague mental images, words, coloured light, faint smells or tastes, strange and indescribable feelings. These are all signs of the initial awakening within you as your senses try to make sense of this feedback you are now paying attention to. An understanding is gleaned through various forms of synaesthesia, which is constantly honed until it makes perfect 'sense'!

How you sense the synaesthesia from your interactions with Jiki, depends on how you 'work' as a person and, because we all work in a unique way, this means discovering your modalities and how these translate to the source dynamics. Some people experience visual synaesthesia while others hear more. You may be a person who feels things or even tends towards aromas and tastes. Once you know what your main synaesthete abilities are, the most conducive method of progressing is to concentrate on those experiences and consciously recognise them. Very often people want to 'see' so much that they ignore the very loud messages they are 'hearing', whereas if they were to concentrate on experiencing those aural messages they would eventually start to sense synaesthesia visually as well.

Intuitive Ability

Your intuition can be described as the way you interpret the feedback you have sensed. So, having recognised your synaesthesia, you need to translate this in some way. Your intuitive skills will enable you to do this, translating the experiences within you into extremely accurate and usable concepts. These, you can then communicate to others or form into insights about the environment around you.

When using your Jiki interactions intuitively to enhance treatments or other areas of your Mastery, you will find that flashes of inspiration or streams of information come to you. However, during your training period, you will need to work on becoming accustomed to Jiki and how it behaves. Translation of the experiences you have is often the most challenging aspect for people learning to work intuitively.

The perspective of Ki is very different to our human perception of the physical world, yet we often interpret things in a very physical way—taking abstract experiences and making them into literal translations. When we encounter any form of intuitive feedback, our subconscious body-mind attempts to translate the information in a way that your conscious mind will understand. Your subconscious works in images and sounds; its linguistic ability is limited to a few words and 'puns'; plus it can only recognise the internal—as far as your subconscious is concerned, only you exist. Every other person in the world is just a part of you!

If you run your synaesthetic experiences through these 'filters', you will often end up with very different results to the things you started with! So whenever you experience synaesthesia, you should always work with that information in the following way:

- Change all 'other people' into aspects of yourself.
- Images either refer to the self, or they will be a play on words.
- 'Inside' (so a car, house, etc.) will mean the body.
- 'Outside' (a landscape, etc.) will refer to expressions of self, beyond the body.
- Images are often symbolic (water is emotion, fire is destruction, air is life, and so on)
- Subconscious translations will refer to your personal experience.

When we first start to investigate our psychic abilities and intuitive thought, we will often perceive 'dream-like' information that is very image based and symbolic. Yet, as we learn how to translate more effectively, it will become an automatic process that can become very elaborate and give huge amounts of detailed information. This not only refers to experiences during treatments, but also in every aspect of life.

Imagination and Descriptive Skills

These skills are another interesting yet often underrated aspect of psychic development and Ki arts as we usually try to divorce our psychic sense from our imagination. The most common piece of feedback given by students is, "But did I imagine it?" The honest answer is—yes, you did!

You are having very real interactions with Ki, interpreting these in an adaptive and intuitive way. While your senses will provide an accurate picture of what is there, your synaesthesia is highly abstract. Thus, it falls to your imagination to translate what you experience synaesthetically. The part of your brain that deals with this translation is also the part that drives your imagination—so in the initial stages of training it does indeed seem like you are imagining it!

However, as we progress and experience more and more, we learn to decipher what is translation and what is 'creation'. We know 'this' is psychic information and 'that' is what we have visualised. It is only with evolution, practice and a belief in yourself that this differentiation comes but, with time and perseverance, it will happen.

The flip side of this is that once you have a workable translation of what you have experienced, how do you convey this to others? It is surprising how difficult it can be to communicate what we perceive in a way that expresses exactly what we feel and that will impart the intricacies of our experiences. Very often it is an inadequacy of our descriptive skills that lets us down, so expansion of our illustrative skills is also a crucial element of psychic ability.

Reading a dictionary (or better still, a thesaurus) is a great way of broadening your vocabulary, especially if you apply the words you learn into everyday conversation. Words around shape, colour, texture, motion, etc., are excellent to have in your linguistic repertoire when finding that exact expression is essential to support others. You may also find that taking up a creative pastime will help you develop magical descriptive skills —it is incredible how much you can learn about colours from oil painting!

Assertion and Confidence

The last phase of vJiki training which is important to the development of your abilities is that of assertion and confidence, which we could view as 'knowing oneself'. Gathering an in-depth knowledge of who you are, will help you to trust yourself with a greater degree of integrity—it will also help you to become unsusceptible to 'external physical influences', which, contrary to popular belief, is more likely to be human in origin as opposed to paranormal!

Assertion is traditionally known as 'protection', but it is much better to use the term 'assertion'. (We only ever protect ourselves from things that are 'unknown', 'bigger than us' or 'uncontrollable'.) By asserting yourself, you will be less likely to undergo entrainment from the physical influences around you. You can, therefore, make the conscious decision as to whether your experiences are conducive to wellbeing or the results you want to achieve. Assertion enables you to interact with Ki, whilst developing your psychic abilities in a way that is positive, empowering and comfortable for you.

Confidence derives from your assertion; the more assertive you are, the more confident you will feel. Confidence is vital to the use of your psychic ability; we need confidence in ourselves and the experiences we have, as well as the confidence to communicate that information to others. By developing our confidence, we not only assist our psychic abilities, but we also evolve in personality and strength of character.

The important element to remember with confidence building is not to let it develop into 'arrogance' or allow it to be dented by the arrogance of others. Confidence is a belief in yourself whereas arrogance is a belief that you are better than others at something. We need confidence to work psychically, but this can have a tendency to develop into the arrogance of believing that we are right and others are wrong.

We all work in our own unique ways and so connect into different perspectives and facets of Ki. When we sense something differently to another person, the idea is to develop the confidence to believe in what you find for yourself, while understanding that the other person's interpretation is equally valid. We should also be aware that if another tells us that they are right and we are wrong, we should be confident enough to stand firm in our abilities and not permit them to dent our belief in those skills.

The Intuition Workout

When attempting to understand how our psychic abilities work, it really helps to have an alternative perspective on the traditional theories. By exploring some of the most recent theories on the physiology of intuition, and how the human body can sense and interact with facets of Ki (that usually fall beyond our sensory range), we can revolutionise our perspective. We discuss these theories at length in the practitioner degree of *The Reiki Revolution Home Experience*, but, as an introduction, let us explore the babbling streams that lead, eventually, to the Falls of Grace and Fountain of Infinite Potential (two regions of the River Realm).

When we refer to the experiences of psychic phenomena and synaesthesia, we are referring to awareness that is based on sensory feedback. However, where is this feedback derived from? What aspects of our senses actually detect the interaction we are having? Is it our fingertips? Or taste buds? Our eyes? Well, just as we use our nervous system to sense other forms of stimuli such as the nerves in our eyes that sense light and the nerves in our ears that sense waves of sound, we use our nerves to pick up on more subtle forms of interaction also.

The area of our nervous system that perceives 'subtle vibrations' or 'Extremely Low Frequency' Energy (ELF), is known as the Perineural system and is formed from the connective tissue that bonds your nerves with the surrounding tissue. Along with other connective tissues, it plays a vital role in the body's natural ability to recover from injury or dis-ease. It does this by sending messages throughout the body; messages contained in vibrations.

So the same process that coordinates your body's ability to communicate for the healing of injury, tissue repair and general 'maintenance', also conducts other vibrations to the brain. We usually ignore these 'quiet' frequencies of energy for the much louder stimuli transmitted via our other 5 senses.

However, you can train yourself to be aware of these whispered messages and interpret them into very complex descriptions.

By improving your sensitivity to your Perineural system, you will find your synaesthesia (and hence, your psychic ability) develops naturally. Thus many of the processes and techniques you study when doing any form of psychic training are usually based upon quietening the body to such an extent that you can sense the vibrations being conducted through the Perineural (and other) connective tissues of the body.

Remember also that the Perineural system is denser in the same places as the rest of your nervous system, so you will feel more in these areas. These include you hands, feet, spine (especially the lower spine) and head. So, whenever you are attempting to improve sensitivity, these are the places to focus upon and the greater the focus, the better the sensitivity!

As we saw earlier, your intuitive abilities are simply how you interpret the synaesthesia you experience. The greater the familiarity you have with interpreting this information (and the more descriptively you can do it), the more intensity you will experience in future. Intuiting what you sense, creates a cycle that enhances your sensitivity, so is an important part of the process of nurturing your psychic abilities. We have so much going on in our heads at any given time that we need to attach importance to the things we want to develop. The better and more elaborately you describe your sensory finding, the more you will pay attention to what you are receiving in the future!!

Very often, the favoured method used to work with intuitive skills is attempting to 'guess' at things intuitively, such as the shapes on cards or the colour of the next car to pass. While these are excellent ways of 'checking your progress' they can really knock your confidence when you are learning, so are not advisable.

A really useful confidence-building method for boosting your intuitive abilities is to work in situations where interpretation is at play. This means that to start with, you do not work with a physical focus, instead, favouring those subjects that require interpretation rather than a single definite answer. The reason for this is that, if you are working on less than 100%

accuracy whilst training (and most mediums are rarely 100% accurate!), you can describe details of a historical place or person that can be verified. Some of these details will be correct, some will be inaccurate and many will be unverifiable. This means that getting some of the details right will boost your confidence whereas if you are guessing the colour of a car, you are either right or wrong; there are no half measures here—and incorrect answers do knock confidence.

Some people might suggest that this takes your intuition to the level where you can just 'guess' and stumble upon some right 'answers' anyway, through 'chance' or 'luck'. The thing is, as you develop your skills, you will decrease your erroneous suggestions to almost zero and the accuracy of your information will increase to a very high level of truth with some unverifiable pieces here and there. This comes from a mixture of experience, knowing how to interpret the sensory information you receive and confidence in yourself.

To help you with this process, here is an intuitive-ability exercise (the first in our Intuition Workout) that can enhance your skills, when used on a daily basis:

1. Stand in the centre of a room in a quiet place where you will not be disturbed for the duration of the exercise. Centre yourself, close your eyes and bring your attention inwards. Turn your attention completely to your breathing, taking long, slow, deep breaths that cause your stomach to expand and chest to move outwards to the sides. Breathe this way until you start to feel relaxed and very calm—if you feel dizzy or light-headed, sit down for a while until you feel better.

2. Now, place your hands out in front of you, palms facing down and start to focus on interacting with Jiki while pushing downwards through the air. When you reach the sensation of a resistance (often described as 'like butter'), 'Sit' your hands on this cushion of Jiki and relax your arms into this resting place. If you wish, you can internally ask the Adventurer Mystic to join you in Avatar State. Many people do find this Mystical support

very useful (visit the Mountain Range for the wisdom of the Mystics).

3. State internally, that you want to experience the 'dynamics that are most relevant to your current circumstance' (or whatever the focus of this exercise may be at the time). Wait for a response. This response should take the form of a slight 'magnetic' pull in your hands. The 'pull' should direct one or both of your hands to the left/right. You may also find this sensation pulling you forward or backward and do be prepared for this with 'soft knees' (slightly bent knees, rather than 'locked' knees). If the pull takes you beyond the comfortable reach of your arms, you can walk slowly in the desired direction.

4. Now, search for changes in your Jiki interactions and continue to explore these fluctuation in experience, until you find an area when you cannot push through the 'resistance' without using muscle effort. Bounce your hands along this sensation until you have a good idea of the boundaries. Then push your hands further into the resistance—if the force is too strong and pushes you back, or resists completely, push your fingertips of your left hand into the barrier, creating a claw with your hand that pierces the dynamic rather than pushing. Here, you are using the movements of your hands to symbolise the underlying interactions between you and the dynamics of Jiki.

5. Once you have done this, ask internally, what 'this' is and then clear your mind as best you can. Allow images, words, feelings, sounds and so on, to fill your mind. You might find it helps at this point to clarify what you perceive by saying aloud your experiences.

6. Upon completing this, come fully back into the room, take a seat and have a moment to compose yourself and make any notes.

Once you have mastered this exercise for 2–3 weeks, progress on to this more advanced technique. Here, we see how it is possible to refine your experience of Jiki dynamics to an even greater level of integrity and use the deeper layers of Jiki wisdom. Hence, preparing to enhance your conscious awareness of Jiki interactions for use in treatment, ritual, and so on. It is advisable to begin with several days of regular HatsuJiHo practice and Calibration to the Jiki Orientation, before embarking on the following routine.

3-Step 'Core State' Jiki Practice

Step One – 20 minutes – Once a day for three weeks (1–3)

1. Sit in a comfortable chair with your feet firmly flat on the floor, your spine straight and your head up. If you wish to play an audio companion, light candles and burn essential oils, this will help create the right ambience required for the exercise.
2. Take a few deep breaths and relax, attempting to release any tension that you are holding. Feel yourself sinking back into the chair yet maintain your straight spine and head up position.
3. Now take your attention to your forehead, lifting your eyes to look at the centre of your forehead, under the closed lids. Keeping this eye position take 6 slow deep breaths, each breath lasting 10 seconds on the inhalation and 10 seconds as you exhale. If you cannot do this, take 12 breaths of 5 seconds for each inhalation and 5 seconds for each exhalation. With each breath, feel yourself lifting upwards as if you are stretching towards the ceiling of the room.
4. Now place your tongue to the roof of your mouth, just behind the teeth and contract your pelvic floor muscles —also known as the HuiYin (GV1/CV1). Relax your eyes while continuing to keep them closed. Start your interaction with the Jiki dynamics.
5. Now imagine that you are looking 'into' your head and all is dark except for a small point in the centre of your head. You might want to imagine this point as a star or

as a ball of energy. As you travel towards the light, you want to hone in on the most central point of your head, so that as you get closer, the point becomes smaller and smaller.

6. Keep this visualisation going for 20 minutes and then come back into the room. If at any time during the exercise you feel as if you are falling backwards, go with the sensation and just allow yourself to float "head over heels" repeatedly.

Step Two – 40 minutes – Once a day for three weeks (4–6)

7. Start the routine as for Step One and then, after 20 minutes, you reach your Core-State and bathe in the light. As you just float here in the light, start to sense the interactions with Jiki all around you, begin by paying attention to your hands, feet, head and then travel into the centre of your body. When you are completely immersed in your experience of Jiki, pay attention to the synaesthesia available to you.

8. Now, get the sense that there is a bubble of light all around you and this bubble contains all the infinite patterns and dynamics that exist. Start to see these "unwrapping", as if you are shedding the surface layers away to reveal what is hidden underneath. Start off with one or two individual dynamics (which you could see as threads or lengths of string, maybe even as 'ethereal onions') and then start to simultaneously unwrap all the dynamics at once, seeing the 'peelings' fall away from you. As you do this, the light gets brighter and brighter; the Jiki interactions, more and more powerful.

9. Continue with this for 20 minutes and then come back into the room.

Step Three – 60 minutes – Once a day for three weeks (7–9)

10. Begin with Steps One and Two, until 40 minutes have elapsed and then continue with the routine as listed below.

11. Floating at the centre of your being (Core-State), unwrapping the dynamics, start to be aware of every single thread/onion/dynamic in existence. Feel each one extending from this central point outwards into the infinite Universe—never-ending, always being.
12. Start to expand outwards along each and every dynamic —reading it, knowing it. Make sure that you expand equally in all directions; taking your time at first to ensure that you are increasing the size of the light bubble in a uniform way, then becoming faster and faster. Decipher every dynamic equally and at the same time—do not focus on any one dynamic.
13. Do this until you recognise the motion/sensation created by travelling along the dynamics and can simply flow with this feeling without thinking about it. Continue this for 20 minutes and then come back into the room.

You will only ever need to complete this 3-Step routine once as, by the time you have completed the 9 weeks, it will be second nature to you.

As soon as you have conducted this exercise for 9 weeks in total, you can then activate the routine very quickly by following the steps below.

1. Lift (closed) eyes to look at forehead
2. Take 5 deep breaths
3. Relax eyes
4. Contract your HuiYin/Place tongue to roof of mouth
5. Begin Jiki interactions
6. Look at centre of head and travel there immediately
7. Imagine all Jiki dynamics flowing out from this point
8. Travel along those dynamics, expanding outwards
9. Come back into room upon completion of treatment

You can use this routine at the start of any vReiki/vJiki treatment, or if providing a psychic reading. You can adapt the part where you are travelling along the dynamics to expand through your client's perspective of the dynamics and gain intuitive knowledge about what is affecting them at any given moment now or in the future (on their present path).

Upon first glance, it may seem that this routine involves a lot of time and effort in the initial stages with 9 weeks of daily practice and in some instances done in parallel with other exercises. However, do bear in mind that this method is really intended for those who wish to enhance the psychic side of their training.

If your interest lies more with the other elements of vReiki practice, then do feel free to leave this routine for the moment, either running through the 9 week programme at a later date, or not at all. It should be mentioned that despite its initial time consumption, this method only requires the initial 9-week process after which you can use it indefinitely.

Appendices

APPENDIX A: KI CULTIVATION TECHNIQUES

HatsuReiHo

vReiki, like so many other techniques, requires practice on a regular basis. You get out what you put in. The Orientations you Calibrate to at each level will offer you a foundation level ability to build upon, although how strong your interactions are for you relies directly on the amount of practice you do. Regular self-treatments and also giving treatments to others will increase the depth of interaction enormously. Also there are techniques from the traditional Usui system of Reiki Mastery collectively called "HatsuReiHo".

The Japanese word "Ho" translates to "Technique" and is often used in Usui Reiki systems. "Hatsu" means "to begin", "to start" or "to Activate" and "Rei" means "Universal Force", "Soul" or "Spirit". So HatsuReiHo could be interpreted as "Start Reiki Technique", or "Soul Activation Technique". Derived from Tendai Buddhism, elements of the HatsuReiHo can be seen in other systems such as meridian massage or QiGong.

In Japan, Usui Reiki training would consist of weekly Reiju Empowerments. These establish a connection to Reiki. HatsuReiHo is then used to intensify that connection and stimulate the meridians of the participant. The routine prompts, encourages and strengthens the interactions with Reiki. It is said that while the ability to connect with Reiki will never fade, the practice of HatsuReiHo, regular Reiju empowerments and also living by the principles of Usui Reiki, ensure a student's development spiritually and as an Usui Reiki therapist.

Many of the elements of HatsuReiHo have various forms, most of which follow an identical theme. As with so many of the general Usui Reiki practices, intention, commitment and confidence are an integral part of the end result and these are the areas that should be focused on rather than getting caught up in the physical procedures. Running through the motions of HatsuReiHo to the letter, but with one eye on the clock, will be nowhere near as effective as carrying out the rough procedure but with heartfelt passion and 100% dedication.

The elements of HatsuReiHo are used at all levels of Usui Reiki practice and will produce optimum results if practised every day for about 10 minutes in the ways described below. Please do remember that, because this is a traditional technique, and to preserve the authenticity of those traditions, archaic concepts, such as 'flow' and 'projection' are used. This is acceptable when working with Usui Reiki, however do be sure not to transition these into the framework of vReiki.

Begin by sitting down and relaxing your body and mind, close your eyes, ensure that your spine is straight and that you are comfortable with good back support. Your feet should be placed firmly on the floor and your hands should be positioned palms down on your lap. Now take your attention down to the Dantien, which is approximately 3 to 5 centimetres below your belly button, and really explore the sensations there while affirming to yourself mentally that you are about to do HatsuReiHo.

Technique: Kenyoku or Dry Bathing

Kenyoku is a cleansing technique and a derivation of the traditional method using ice-cold water! It can be viewed as a way of brushing away contractive experiences, to detach oneself from a client or situation, and to clear the mind of stray thoughts. This is an excellent way of bringing you into the present time and invoking a state of "living in the moment".

There are numerous ways of performing Kenyoku; these are some of the most extensively practised:

Dr Usui's Traditional Technique

Stage One: Place your right hand on your left collarbone, with the palm flat against your chest then, in one continuous motion, bring your hand down across your chest and down to the right hip. Do the same motion, but using your left hand on the right shoulder. Complete this stage by repeating the first motion, beginning with right hand on left shoulder.

Stage Two: Using the right hand, stroke from the left wrist across the palm and out past the fingers of the left hand. Do this movement again reversing your hands (left hand brushing right hand) and then repeat the original action (right hand brushing left hand).

1st Modern Version

Stage One: Place your right hand on your left collarbone with the palm flat against your chest then, in one continuous motion, bring your hand down across your chest and down to the right hip. Do the same motion again but using your left hand on the right shoulder. Complete this stage by repeating the first motion beginning with your right hand on your left shoulder.

Stage Two: Position your right hand on your left shoulder with your left arm slightly outstretched and palm facing down. Stroke the outside of the arm down the entire length then continue across the left hand and out past the fingers. Do this again using your left hand on your right shoulder and then once again with your right hand and your left shoulder.

2nd Modern Version

Stage One: Place your right hand on your left collarbone with the palm flat against your chest then, in one continuous motion, bring your hand down across your chest and down to the right hip. Do the same motion again using your left hand on the right shoulder. Complete this stage by repeating the first motion beginning with your right hand on your left shoulder.

Stage Two: Position the index and middle finger of your right hand on your left shoulder with your left arm flat against your body. Brush down the outside of the arm continuing down to the left hip and then out away from the body. Do this again using your left hand on your right shoulder and then once again with your right hand and your left shoulder.

A Variation

Stage One: Place your right hand on your left collarbone with the palm flat against your chest then, in one continuous motion, bring your hand down across your chest and down to the right hip. Do the same motion again using your left hand on the right shoulder. Complete this stage by repeating the first motion beginning with your right hand on your left shoulder.

Stage Two: With the right hand, place your palm flat against the collarbone of the left shoulder and, with your left arm outstretched, brush down the inside of the left arm then across the wrist, palm and out past the fingers of the left hand. Repeat once with opposite hand and shoulder and then a third time with the left shoulder/right hand.

Experiment with each of the above and find the one that offers the best results for you.

Technique: Connection to Reiki

With your hands raised high in the air, palms to the zenith and fingers pointing directly behind you, connect to the force of Reiki. You can do this by visualising white light or feeling the sensation of a surge down into your palms and flowing down your arms and into your body. As you become aware of the sensations you may feel your arms begin to lower. If you do not feel this, start to lower them anyway. Bring your arms out to the sides 'pulling' the light around you as if you are creating a bubble that encapsulates you. Bring the light past your crown and into your body, holding the interaction at your Dantien point (around the belly button area—visit The Waterfall for more information). Then pull your arms down and around to meet on your lap, palms facing the Dantien and your dominant hand closer to the skin.

Technique: Joshin Kokkyu Ho or Purifying the Spirit

With your hands still on your lap, palms positioned towards your Dantien, focus on the interactions that are here. Now place your tongue against the roof of your mouth just behind the top set of teeth and contract the HuiYin (pelvic floor muscles). Breathe in deeply; drawing the air down into your lower back and allow your stomach to rise and your chest to expand to the sides. Visualise the light flooding in through your crown and down to your Dantien, gathering there with each in-breath.

Now, as you exhale, allow your tongue to fall, relax your HuiYin and feel the light flowing out from your Dantien, travelling vigorously from your palms and fingers, your feet and toes. Then repeat the process by inhaling as you did above. You can continue with this technique as long as you like, or is comfortable for you. However, if you begin to feel light headed or faint, stop immediately. This technique should be used with caution by those with high blood pressure or in the latter stages of pregnancy.

Technique: Gassho Meiso or The Gassho Meditation

The translation of Gassho means 'two hands coming together' and is achieved by placing your hands together as if praying and positioned just above the heart centre. A good way of checking if you have the right positioning on the hands is to gently breathe out through the nose and you should be able to feel the breath on your fingertips. Whilst maintaining this position, remember to breathe using the Joshin Kokkyu Ho technique unless the contraindications already stated suggest otherwise.

Become aware of the place between your middle fingertips. Focus on that space and completely clear your mind of all else. You may find this very hard at first but as each new thought comes into your awareness, just acknowledge it and send it away very calmly then bring your attention back to the place where your middle fingers touch. The more you do this, the more you will learn to just 'be': not only a valuable state for Reiki practice, but also an incredible state for spiritual enlightenment.

This is the position you should maintain when receiving Reiju empowerments

Gokai Sansho or Reflecting on the Usui Reiki Principles

This is an optional part of HatsuReiHo, however it can be very grounding to remind yourself of the principles and this enables you to place them into your personal outlook and daily life. Say to yourself either mentally or out loud:

Just for today...
>...Do not anger
>...Do not worry
>...Be thankful
>...Endeavour in work
>...Nurture dharma for all your teachers
>...Be kind to all living things

Place your hands back on your lap with your palms down. Say to yourself internally that you have completed HatsuReiHo and give thanks, before opening your eyes, wiggling your toes and shaking your hands; so coming back fully into the room.

HatsuJiHo

HatsuJiHo is based on the traditional Usui Reiki technique of HatsuReiHo, with some added elements that will help increase the effectiveness of your Jiki practice.

1. From a seated position, place your right hand on your left collarbone with the palm flat against your chest then, in one continuous motion, bring your hand down across your chest and down to the right hip. Do the same motion but using your left hand on the right shoulder. Complete this stage by repeating the first motion, beginning with your right hand on your left shoulder.

2. Using the right hand, stroke from the left wrist down across the palm and out past the fingers of the left hand. Do this movement again but reversing hands (left hand brushing right hand) and then repeat the original action (right hand brushing left hand).

3. Hold your arms outstretched to the sides with your palms at 90 degrees to your arms so that they are facing the walls on either side. Breathe deeply and try to feel the Jiki flowing into one hand and repelling the other. With each slow in-breath, pull the Jiki through one hand and, as you breathe out, push the Jiki away with the other.

4. Now slowly bend your arms at the elbow and swing your forearm/hands to the front of your body at chest height. Now hold your hands in this position, facing away from you, until they begin to move into the Gassho position (praying hands).

5. Then place your tongue against the roof of your mouth just behind the top set of teeth and contract the HuiYin. Breathe in deeply; drawing the air into your lower back, allowing your stomach to rise and chest to expand to the sides. Visualise sparks of light at your crown and in your heart area, becoming more vibrant with each in-breath.

6. As you exhale, allow your tongue to fall, relax your HuiYin and feel your entire body begin to glow, scanning each part of your body with your attention and increasing the level of interaction with Jiki at that place, before moving to the next. Then repeat the process by inhaling, as above. You can continue with this technique as long as you like, or is comfortable. However, if you begin to feel light headed or faint, stop immediately.

7. With practice, you should begin to feel a circular motion within you, rather like a vortex of energy. This sensation is often very magnetic and can be very powerful. Allow the spinning to happen faster and faster until you find a place of complete stillness and peace (akin to the eye of the storm), even though the vortex is gyrating very quickly.
8. Now, keeping your stillness, try to sense the Jiki within you; attempting not to connect to the rapid motion, but perceiving the gentle patterns that are created from it. This is a little like looking out of the window from a car that is travelling at speed—all is blurred except for an occasional shape or flash of some image.
9. Now start to focus upon the Jiki dynamics that you want in your life, the loving relationship, the healthy lifestyle, the prosperous business, the friends and family and so on. As you do this, dissolve the dynamics you do not want in your life such as the stresses and strains, the never-ending bills, the health issues, the arguments, etc.
10. Rest your hands down onto your lap; palms down. Say to yourself internally that you have completed HatsuJiHo and give thanks, before opening your eyes, wiggling your toes and shaking your hands; coming back fully into the room.

This technique can be done every day or interspersed with HatsuReiHo practice. You may also choose to combine the two techniques, working through the dry bathing, connection to Reiki, Dantien Breathing, Connection to Jiki, Jiki Vortex, and finally Gassho principles/meditation.

APPENDIX B: USUI REIKI TREATMENT METHODS

The Self-Treatment

In Usui Reiki practice, a distinction is made between self-healing and the treatment of others although it is widely thought that by working on other people, the practitioner also gains the benefits of the treatment also. In Usui Reiki, regular self-treatment was seen as a necessary part of the practice and a way of intensifying the healing benefits afforded by Reiki. Essential in the first few weeks after Reiju Empowerment, the self-treatment can help the body to detoxify quicker, thus smoothing the Energy Alignment Process (EAP) and ensuring clearer interactions with Reiki.

The traditional routine for conducting a self-treatment is as follows, although it is just as worthwhile to go to sleep at night with your hands on your chest or stomach. By simply ensuring that you interact with Reiki before going to sleep, you will be treated while you sleep! Remember that you do not need to allot hours of your daily routine to self-treatment, you can incorporate your treatment into meditation, whilst sitting on a bus or train, even while watching TV!

Degree One Treatment of Others

Once you have experienced your Reiju Empowerment, you will be able to interact with Reiki immediately and the first method of treating others is a simple set of 'hand positions' that you can use to give structure to your practice. The important thing to remember with hand positions is that the interaction between you and Reiki will occur wherever it needs to; the hand positions simply offer structure to a treatment (visit The Temple to see the hand position charts).

A full Reiki treatment will normally last for about an hour. You should spend about 4–5 minutes in each of the hand positions, but if you can feel a lot of Ki in your hands then you can hold that position for longer: a lot longer if you feel it is necessary. The best results are obtained when you are calm and relaxed so becoming at one with the energy. If you are giving a treatment while having an animated conversation with someone, you will not create the most intense interactions possible.

When you have had some regular practice in treating other people, your Reiki interactions will begin to guide your body to different areas of your client, suggesting where treatment is most needed. This is an excellent sign that your intuition is developing and can be enhanced even further by progressing to the next treatment style.

Reiji Ho and Byosen Reikan Ho

In addition to the traditional hand positions, techniques that play an integral part of Usui Reiki training, are the Japanese scanning techniques: Byosen Reikan Ho and Reiji Ho. Usually taught as part of the first degree training in Japan, these techniques are occasionally offered as part of Usui Reiki 2 in the Westernised Reiki systems, yet are mostly omitted despite their traditional importance and treatment effectiveness.

Separately these two techniques enable you to increase the sensitivity to areas where the interactions with Ki are vague or stagnating. By using your hands and body, you can develop your intuitive ability by interpreting and understanding the movements you experience. Byosen Reikan Ho is used to monitor disruptions (known as 'Byosen') in the Ki that a person is expressed through. Once detected, these can be dissolved or reduced to enable healthy Ki interactions throughout the body. By conducting regular and long-term Byosen Reikan Ho practice with many different people, it is possible to develop a very refined skill in intuitive sensitivity.

Traditionally, Byosen are associated with a person's disease, illness or injury and can be felt in the hands of the practitioner. The sensation (also known as 'Hibiki' or 'resonance') will depend on the variety, source and strength of the Byosen, but a common description is of an insect crawling across the skin or a small coil springing across the practitioner's hand. Other Hibiki include pain, numbness, heat, coldness, tickling, tingling, etc.

Byosen are said to appear a few days before the symptoms develop and may still be present after the dis-ease has passed, which can mean that a person may develop the symptoms again. This denotes that even if your treatment subject is in 'perfect health', they still may have Byosen associated with potential dis-ease. This does also imply that you can also treat the Byosen to stop the dis-ease from ever (re)appearing.

What you actually feel with each Hibiki will depend on the cause and status of the dis-ease and the time it will take to heal. The presence of a Byosen in a specific location does not necessarily mean that the dis-ease is positioned in the same physical area as each Byosen may actually appear in a completely different place from the actual symptom. What is important when sensing the Byosen is to relax, clear your mind and work with each Byosen in detail, really trying to hone in on the sensations in your hand.

Whilst Byosen Reikan Ho is a cerebral activity that requires the conscious scanning of your treatment subject, Reiji Ho is conducted in a completely intuitive way. As the practitioner, you do not need to be aware of the dis-ease or issue and its relevant treatment, as the entire process is completed intuitively. Reiji Ho comes naturally to some people and takes plenty of practice with others. It is often found that people who instinctively take to Reiji Ho, find mastering Byosen Reikan Ho a challenging experience and vice versa, although this is not always the case. Regardless of the natural ability in either technique, both Reiji Ho and Byosen Reikan Ho are cornerstones of Reiki tradition that require regular practice to be mastered.

Byosen Reikan Ho

To conduct a treatment using Byosen Reikan Ho, simply start by interacting with Reiki via a 'head connection': this is when you place your hands either side of your subject's head and shift your perspective to an interaction between you, your client, and Reiki. Then use your non-dominant hand to 'scan' your subject's body, sensing the Hibiki of Byosen in the area surrounding the body. Upon discovering a Byosen, interact with Reiki while focusing upon the location. Continue this until the Hibiki has ceased or 10 minutes have passed.

Upon dissolving the Byosen, repeat the scanning process until you have located and cleared as many Byosen as possible in the treatment time. Complete the treatment with a final head connection and then bring your treatment subject back into the room.

Reiji Ho

To conduct a Reiji Ho treatment, simply start with a head connection and state internally that you are going to treat your subject with Reiji Ho. When you experience a strong interaction with Reiki, move to the side of your subject and place your hands over their abdominal region. Continue to interact with Reiki until your hands begin to move to a new position; allow this to happen. It is important not to make a change happen, or resist the movement when it does—just go with it! This could be seen as you twisting into a new perspective and using your body to synaesthetically guide you.

If your hands move to their fullest extent, feel free to travel around your subject to obtain a more comfortable position for yourself. Remain at each position until your hands once again move of their own accord. This can look rather like the gentle movement and positions of TaiChi or Qigong! At the end of the treatment go to your subject's head area and finish with a head connection.

To explore these treatment methods further, please visit the virtual Realms, especially, the Temple and The Waterfall areas.

OTHER vREIKI BOOKS IN THE REIKI REVOLUTION HOME EXPERIENCE:

This book is part of *The Reiki Revolution Home Experience* from mPowr; a multi-sensory and immersive journey that enables you to become completely enchanted with your studies in an engaging and compelling way. To enrol on your vReiki adventure, simply visit the mPowr website.

vReiki Two: The Reiki Revolution Practitioner

vReiki Two: The Fountain & The Tree (eBook)

vReiki Three: Mentoring the Reiki Revolution

vReiki Four: Mastering the Reiki Revolution

BOOKS AND VAEOS FROM THE AUTHOR:

The Key: To Business and Personal Success

Legacy VAEO

Bedtime Stories from the Woodland

AUDIO PROGRAMMES FROM THE AUTHOR:

Synaesthesia Symphony Live

Synaesthesia Symphony V:The Harmonies of Health

The PsyQ Orientation

FOR FURTHER INFORMATION PLEASE VISIT:

www.mpowrpublishing.com and www.celtic-reiki.com

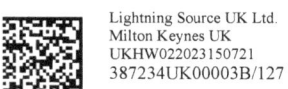

Lightning Source UK Ltd.
Milton Keynes UK
UKHW022023150721
387234UK00003B/127